PRIMARY NURSING

Nursing in the Burford and Oxford
Nursing Development Units

Edited by
ALAN PEARSON MSc, PhD, SRN

Professor and Dean of Nursing,
Deakin University,
Geelong,
Victoria,
Australia

CHAPMAN & HALL
London · Glasgow · New York · Tokyo · Melbourne · Madras

Published by Chapman & Hall, 2-6 Boundary Row, London SE1 8HN

Chapman & Hall, 2-6 Boundary Row, London SE1 8HN, UK

Blackie Academic & Professional, Wester Cleddens Road, Bishopbriggs, Glasgow G64 2NZ, UK

Chapman & Hall, 29 West 35th Street, New York NY10001, USA

Chapman & Hall Japan, Thomson Publishing Japan, Hirakawacho Nemoto Building, 6F, 1-7-11 Hirakawa-cho, Chiyoda-ku, Tokyo 102, Japan

Chapman & Hall Australia, Thomas Nelson Australia, 102 Dodds Street, South Melbourne, Victoria 3205, Australia

Chapman & Hall India, R. Seshadri, 32 Second Main Road, CIT East, Madras 600 035, India

First edition 1988
Reprinted 1988, 1989, 1991, 1992

© 1988 Alan Pearson

Printed in Great Britain by The Ipswich Book Company, Ipswich

ISBN 0 412 34070 4

A catalogue record for this book is available from the British Library
Library of Congress Cataloging-in-Publication Data available

Table of Contents

Preface

The nursing development unit established in Burford in 1981, and its sister unit opened in Oxford in 1985, have from their beginnings tried to implement and evaluate a professional focus on nursing practice. Using only qualified nurses in the delivery of care, and developing a system of primary nursing, the units have tried to emphasise the therapeutic role of nursing, and the need to establish hospital beds specifically for patients with nursing problems.

In many ways, little has been achieved. There are still many problems in trying to work in a way which is, to some of us, quite alien to our initial nurse training; the new system is plagued with criticism from others outside the unit; and there is still the nagging doubt of 'are we going along the right road?' which is inevitable in an environment that encourages a questioning attitude. However, if all was well, it was thought that we had got it right and nursing in the units was perfect, complacency would set in, and there would be no need to improve and develop.

So, in some ways, perhaps something has been achieved. The introduction of a new care team structure and the enhancement of the role of the direct caregiving nurse has been successful, and nursing beds have been established and are being objectively evaluated. More importantly, the units have actively and deliberately published widely on the issues being grappled with, and run a large number of study days and courses for nurses and other health care workers. Even if the result of this is sometimes criticism of the unit's philosophy, nevertheless the issues have been brought to the fore in nursing circles. The purpose of this book is to present, in one volume, the underlying beliefs, fundamental principles, and practical realities of using a system of primary nursing in hospitals, and of establishing nursing beds in the health care system. All of the contributors work in the development unit and have clinical roles.

We believe in the need for two major initiatives if nursing is to have its full healing potential released:

● the introduction of the sort of nursing practice we describe here in *all* inpatient settings;

● the establishment of a nursing unit in every hospital or health service neighbourhood.

A most ambitious and perhaps impossible dream, but as Tiny Tim said:
'Dreaming is better than parties.'

Alan Pearson
Burford
Oxfordshire

Contributors

Angela Wharton SRN, Primary Nurse, Burford Community Hospital

Richard McMahon SRN, Nurse Practitioner, Oxford Nursing Development Unit

Plaxy-Anita Muetzel BSc, RGN, Formerly Associate Nurse, Oxford Nursing Development Unit

Steven Ersser BSc, SRN, Associate Nurse, Oxford Nursing Development Unit

1

Trends in Clinical Nursing

Alan Pearson

INTRODUCTION

In the last 20 years, much radical thinking has emerged in nursing, and it has been a time of much exhortation to change, even though the practical evidence of this at the patient's bedside is often disappointing. As in most practice disciplines, there seems to be a rather wide — and gloomy — gap between the ideas of the leaders, educators and thinkers, and the reality of the world of the practitioner. 'Why,' say the former, 'won't they change,' and 'How,' say the latter, 'can we with so much to do, so many obstacles, and so little help?' Both this chapter and the next discuss these ideas of the 'thinkers' — the trends in nursing that cannot happen until they are actually taken on board in practice. Subsequent chapters discuss how they are being interpreted and implemented in a place where real patients are nursed by real nurses.

NURSING TODAY

Nurses are present in all areas of the health care system — in hospitals, in the community, and within general practice, and '. . . are present at the birth and death of most of us and could be considered the worker bees of the system' (Tiffany, 1977). The role of the nurse, however, remains unclear, and there are still no widely accepted views on what nursing is, who should nurse, and when and where (McFarlane, 1980). Furthermore, despite nurses constituting the largest occupational group in the health service, they make little contribution to decision-making, and are in fact seen as being subservient to medicine (Friedson, 1975). As long as the system revolves around the medical model of:

$$\text{Diagnosis} \longrightarrow \text{Treatment} \longrightarrow \text{Cure}$$

(McFarlane, 1980) nursing will continue to be subservient, and play a less than satisfactory role in decision-making in terms of client need. There is growing evidence that nursing does concentrate on such a model; that it operates in a highly routinised way; and that it resists patient involvement, encouraging patient conformity to the established rules.

McFarlane (1980) says that it is possible to argue: '. . . that the caring role of the nurse has been so neglected that this needs expansion (in depth) and that the nursing model of care needs to be more developed: ie

$$\text{Assessment} \longrightarrow \text{Help} \longrightarrow \text{Self-care.'}$$

(of self-care   (assistance etc)
disabilities)

THE NEED FOR CHANGE

As is typical of all organised occupations, nursing has been exhorted to change by its leaders at least since the emergence of Florence Nightingale over a century ago! Contemporary leaders still urge nurses enthusiastically to pursue changes to reflect current trends. For the last 20 years, there has been emphasis on the need to move away from the established pattern of practice based on routinisation, allocation of tasks and adherence to management and medical models, to a pattern based on meeting the individual needs of the consumer, and to focusing on professionaling the nursing role to allow for autonomous practice.

Davies (1976) suggests that in nursing physical care is ranked above psychosocial care, and this has become subject to rule following, standardised activity and a clear nursing hierarchy with firm allocation of supervisory responsibility. The literature supports this view and offers some explanations.

Such standardisation is an effective way of avoiding some of the stress and anxiety inherent in the nurses' work and helps to maintain 24 hour cover when facing high staff turnover and assimilating part-time staff. The pervasive routinisation in clinical care is partly, suggests Menzies (1960), a social defence system set up by hospital nursing services 'to protect its members against the stress arising from their work'.

Rigid routines are imposed to remove the need for stressful decision-making and nursing schools socialise students into valuing routine and in performing their role in an impersonal manner without creative thought or attempting to solve problems. Most nursing schools, suggests Stein (1978), are highly disciplined, inculcate subservience and inhibit deviance. A fear of independent action results, and clinging to hierarchical support systems becomes a needed and appreciated activity.

Davies (1977) points out how the heavy reliance on nurses as teachers, and the protection of student nurses from external influences, acts as a strong and effective socialisation influence to preserve routinisation. It transforms current work practices into valued work practices and removes a great deal of uncertainty from the work.

Patients themselves agree with the view that nurses are obsessed with the performance of tasks associated with physical care and the support of medical regimes and that they do not fulfil expectations as the humanisers of the health care system. Cartwright (1964), Spelman, Ley and Jones (1966), and Raphael (1969) all report large numbers of patients included in their studies mentioning communication problems (61 per cent, 44 per cent and 86 per cent respectively). Reynolds (1978) found considerable dissatisfaction about information received in general surgical wards, and Eardley et al. (1975) found that education for patients with chronic disability was regarded as totally inadequate. Stockwell (1972) reports that patients involved in her study would have liked more opportunities to talk with nurses but knew they were 'too busy'. Nursing is criticised by patients studied by the Royal Commission on the National Health Service (1979): 88 per cent of patients regarding paramedical workers as being 'considerate' to them as individuals; 84 per cent for ancillary workers, but only 80 per cent for nurses.

Duberley (1977) argues strongly that carrying out both medical orders and routine are highly valued, and that British nursing generally offers a service based largely on medical diagnosis, the 'consultant's and/or ward sister's preference', and the ward routine for each ward.

3

Kratz (1977) acknowledges that ward sisters attempt to plan care, but the plan is based chiefly on doctors' notes, what the patient says in conversation, and the added hospital routines, such as 'BD — TPRs, early morning tea and no washing of legs on Sundays (because of staff shortages)'.

The subservience of clinical nurses to both doctors and nurses in management positions is well documented in the literature. Since the beginning of this century nursing has been firmly linked with medicine and largely based in institutions (Mayers, 1972). The historical growth of nursing has led to an adoption of the belief that the role of the nurse is to help the doctor (Beyers and Phillips, 1971; Wiedenbach, 1964). The massive expansion of hospital care systems that began in the 1920s furthered this view of nursing, and the growth in medical technology demanded the development of a group of workers subservient to the doctors who would apply and monitor this technology and be the doctor's 'eyes and ears' (Pavey, 1954). The focus of nursing became the same as that of medicine — to cure (Goffman, 1968) — and nurses strove to keep patients in a disadvantaged infantile position and thus dependent (Miller and Gwynne, 1972).

In areas where cure was not probable, such as long-term care units, the problematic results of nursing adhering to the medical model became apparent because care was positioned at the bottom of a vertical continuum with cure at the top. Miller and Gwynne (1972) postulate a 'warehouse model' which is, in effect, a hospital model imposed on those whose needs cannot be appropriately met by applying the medical model. It involves 'people processing' where cure is reinterpreted to mean the 'postponement of death as long as possible'.

The routine work, subordinate to the work of the doctors, needed to be organised and supervised (Beyers and Phillips, 1971). As the major setting for nursing practice became a bureaucratically structured organisation, linked with nursing's military and religious roots, obedience, discipline and loyalty became emphasised characteristics of the work. The general trends in organisation theory advanced by the proponents of the classical management school filtered into nursing, and facets of 'scientific management' were adopted; this saw the organisation as a machine demanding that everything should be run in an orderly fashion (Perrow, 1965). Although this approach began to lose favour in the light of the emergence of the human relations management school in the 1930s, and later the behaviourally inclined political science view, the highly structured organisation advanced by the 'scientific school' has remained an intrinsic part of nursing.

The literature thus supports the view that all is not well in nursing (and the health care delivery system as a whole). Nurses' leaders use such evidence to persuade nurses that they need to change, and to argue for specific changes.

WHAT NEEDS CHANGING?

McFarlane (1980) asserts that the cure-oriented/medical-oriented model, pervasive routinisation, and a rigid supervisory structure are inappropriate to nursing in any setting and that the needs of individuals are not being met. Many nurses support this and give voice to the view that nurses should move from a medical model of practice to a model conceived for nursing through the analysis of what people need when they are ill, dependent, or unable to perceive how to achieve health. The recognition by many of the need to reform society's beliefs on the role of women led to a questioning of the subservience of nurses (mainly women) to doctors (mainly men), and the criticism by social theorists of the power of medicine (Friedson, 1975; Zola, 1975; Szasz and Hollender, 1975). Nurses began to assert themselves and seek equality within the health care team. Batchelor (1980) lists a number of factors leading to this demand for equality: the changing status of women in society as a whole; the higher status of nurses as reflected by salaries; the enhanced quality of the entry to nurse training; the women's liberation movement; the 'too cosy paternalism' of some doctors; the introduction of a new management structure in nursing; improvement in the quality of nurse training; the increased number of men in senior positions; and the rise in trade union involvement by nurses.

Much of this drive for change in nursing is largely emanating from nurses in leadership positions at national level, and those who became academics after nursing departments were established in the institutes of higher learning in the 1960s (White, 1982). The national nursing bodies exhort nurses to bring about fairly radical practice change based on:

● reorganising work patterns so that care is given by trained nurses, and where accountability to the patient is explicit (Marram, 1979; Pearson, 1983; Binnie, 1984);

● restructuring the nursing team so that the hierarchy is 'flattened' (Gonzalez, 1981);

● developing a close relationship between nurse and patient, and involving the patient in planning care (Hall, 1964; Alfano, 1971; Marriner, 1979);

● basing practice on a model for nursing which incorporates the concept of holism (Smuts, 1926), and clarifies the contribution of nursing to health care (Orem, 1980; Roper, Logan and Tierney, 1981; Pearson and Vaughan, 1984b)

● using a problem-solving approach (Yura and Walsh, 1973; Kratz, 1977; Marriner, 1979; McFarlane and Castledine, 1982).

The amalgamation of these concepts is said to constitute a major reform in nursing (Pearson and Vaughan, 1984b); it is often referred to as the 'nursing process' by a vast array of nursing theorists, and written about frequently in all the major nursing journals. It can be said to represent the current ideology of nursing held by nursing leadership, and implementing it in practice has become the concern of a number of initiatives by policy-making bodies.

However, much criticism has been raised both from the nursing establishment, by articles in the popular nursing press, and from the medical establishment by individual doctors (Mitchell, 1984). Mitchell, in particular, savagely attacks the growing acceptance of the 'new' ideology, claiming that the concepts are 'jargonistic, American imports', and that nurses are attempting to 'progressively exclude doctors from nursing affairs'. Rowden (1984) answers Mitchell's criticisms by offering a patient's perspective; conceding that nurses must involve other members of the health care team, he suggests that perhaps doctors could consult nurses when they anticipate practice change.

Duberley (1977) reports strong resistance by nurses to the suggested changes, because they challenge 'the type of care that nurses generally provide for their patients', and mean 'that accepted practice should be changed'; thus years of past practice is judged as bad and valueless. Mitchell (1984) asserts that the new ideology should not be promoted until there is evidence to support its usefulness and suggests that the patient's opinion should be the one sought. Such evidence is in small supply, with Meyer (1981) reporting some improvement in care of the elderly when problem-solving and allocation of patients to nurses is introduced, and Metcalfe (1982) reporting significantly higher patient satisfaction with care indices in a maternity area where the 'new' ideas were incorporated into practice. Although advice on how to introduce change appears in the literature, accounts of it being implemented appear only rarely, and there is little published evidence to suggest that the new ideology will have a favourable effect on either patient outcomes, or on the satisfaction of nurses.

INTRODUCING THE NEW TRENDS IN NURSING

Changing the focus of nursing towards the individual needs of the patient, based on an alternative to the medical model, involving a change in the nurse/patient relationship, and using a systematic approach to practice is likely to cause major conflict with the traditional ideology of nursing.

Models for practice

The basic curriculum for registered general nurses is still largely based on a medical model, focusing on body systems and disease modes. Davis (1975) argues that nurses receive a 'watered-down' medical training, and that they exit training as substandard doctors; there is much evidence that nurses value carrying out medical procedures and assisting doctors by carrying out 'routine' tasks (MacGuire, 1980). The Royal College of Nursing (1980, 1981) and Orem (1980) argue that the patient will be better served if doctors pursue a medical model approach, concentrating on physiological homeostasis and the diagnosis and treatment of disease/illness, and nurses concentrate on the patient as a person, by helping him/her to make sense of what is happening and giving support and guidance. Alfano (1971) describes how nurses working to the medical model interpret the doctor to the patient, whereas patients themselves wish for the nurse to translate the patient to the doctor. She argues that this demands a reorientation towards a different view of the world of the patient — a model developed for nursing.

7

The drive towards being more specific about the nature of nursing, and to construct models that accurately describe its practice, is therefore decried by both nurses and doctors, yet it has much to recommend it. The difficulty in actually applying models and changing practice is perhaps the major reason for this rejection, rather than logical and rational reasoning.

The most widely known attempt to define nursing is that of Henderson (1966).

The unique function of the nurse is to assist the individual, sick or well, in the performance of those activities contributing to health or its recovery (or to a peaceful death) that he would perform unaided if he had the necessary strength, will or knowledge, and to do this in such a way as to help him gain independence as rapidly as possible.

Many other definitions have been suggested. Bower (1972) sees nursing as 'the application of knowledge to promote and maintain maximum health, comfort and care'. She also points out that the uniqueness of nursing is its property of being able to operate in a highly generalistic manner. Travelbee (1971) expands on this generalistic function and stresses the fact that the nurse is there with the patient 24 hours a day.

The contemporary acceptance of a humanistic approach is reflected in most of the stated definitions, and nursing is often seen as an essentially social activity. As such, the importance of developing relationships — both between nurse and patient, and nurse and co-health workers — is often central. Chapman (1979) proposes that nursing is a 'social activity, an interactive process between individuals, the nurse and the patient', while Sundeen *et al.* (1976) see the nurse as 'being involved with all the components of a person in a dynamic interaction'. La Monica (1979) says that the goal of nursing is 'to provide humanistic care adapted to individual needs'. Thus, contemporary nursing theory seems to be asserting that nursing involves seeing the recipient as a holistic being, and using this view to meet his or her individual needs through meaningful interaction.

Roper (1976) purports that it is not possible to describe adequately what nursing is in a crisp, concise definition. She says that only a broad schematic explanation of an interpretation of what nursing someone entails, presented in the form of a conceptual model, can give meaning to the reality of nursing. Some nurses reject any moves to impose rigid definitions in nursing on its practitioners; McFarlane (1976) concurs with this, suggesting, however, that models are 'conceptual representations of reality', of use in developing nursing as a human service, and Reilly (1975) argues that they are essential to give nurses 'a perspective, a way of looking at nursing'.

McFarlane (1976) argues that all nurses should practise from a knowledge base which is sufficient to enable them to justify the actions they take, and that 'professional' nurses should base practice on a conceptual model. The discussion of developing nursing models is plagued with confusion in the literature. McFarlane (1976) comments on the 'utter semantic confusion' in theorising in nursing, suggesting that it is 'doubtful if clarity can be restored'. Citing Dickoff and James (1968), she observes that nursing grasps at 'concrete, structural security too soon', and asserts that 'like the world of the infant, the world of theory in nursing seems a "blooming, buzzing confusion" '.

Johnson and Davis (1975) describe a conceptual model for nursing practice as a 'systematically constructed, scientifically based, and logically related set of concepts which identify the essential components of nursing practice together with the values required in their use by the practitioner'. This 'diagram', as it were, of what nursing is, provides for the nurse a diagnostic and treatment orientation for the specific practice of nursing (Reihl and Roy, 1980). The 'diagnosis and treatment' refers to *nursing*, and not to the acts of medicine. Reihl and Roy (1980) suggest that the current development of nursing models is a serious attempt to provide alternatives to the disease/medical/hospital-oriented models of the past, and say that contemporary nursing needs to develop models specific to nursing for the patients' sake. They assert that in using the 'nursing process' (Yura and Walsh, 1973) as a means to deliver nursing care, nurses have need of a conceptual model on which to base assessment, identification of patient problems, planning care, implementing care, and evaluation of the outcomes.

Orem (1980) suggests that if nurses use the concepts and theories inherent in a model, they will practise more effectively, and will be able to 'place in perspective other descriptions of nursing including those in other areas of specialisation'. Thus she, along with Roper (1976) believes that a satisfactory model will describe nursing in any context, and will have meaning to

9

nurses in all specialities. Orem (1980) goes on to observe that, through the emergence of models specifically for nursing, the nurse's role is

> emerging from obscurity imposed by an overemphasis on the relationship between the physician and the nurse, and between the employing institution and the nurse . . . Nurses are coming to recognise that an item of information about a patient may have one meaning for a physician, but quite a different meaning for the nurse.

A number of models are described in the literature, and an attempt is made by Reihl and Roy (1980) to construct a unified model for nursing by amalgamating a variety of models. In their classification of nursing models developed to date, they suggest that three types emerge: systems models; developmental models; and interactionist models. In the first two sessions on models with the group, systems models were discussed. The basic premise of those nurses who favour a systems approach is the concept of an open system within an open system. Byrne and Thompson (1978) recommend that man be understood in the context of the subordinate systems of which he is composed, such as cell, organ, and organ systems, and the superordinate systems in which he exists — the family, the community, the society.

Those nursing models which follow systems theory utilise the concept of man as an organism, existing in a steady state, being subjected to stress, and then adapting or adjusting in order to re-establish its stability within the acceptable parameters. Orem (1980) and Roper, Logan and Tierney (1980) both place extra emphasis on development and interaction and, although systems based, expand the conceptualisation outside the narrower confines set by those theorists who attempt to pursue a purist systems approach.

Roper (1976, 1979), and Roper, Logan and Tierney (1980, 1981, 1983) describe a model that incorporates many of the concepts inherent in both the model described by Orem (1980) and the concept outlined by Henderson (1966). Roper, Logan and Tierney's (1980) model for nursing is based on a model for living, and attempts to describe the reality of nursing to help nurses develop a mode of thinking about the profession which focuses on the process of living. Developed from the findings of a research study into clinical experience for student nurses (Roper, 1976), the purpose of the model is to develop nursing as a discipline. Wilson (1972) purports that disciplines are 'forms of thought that have a characteristic approach to appropriate questions related to a subject'. Roper (1976) suggests that the use of a model will allow nurses to think 'nursologically' — that is, in a way characteristic to nursing, in the same way as mathematicians think mathematically, and theologians theologically.

Roper, Logan and Tierney's model for nursing identifies the subject of nursing as the individual, seeing him as a person engaged in living through his lifespan. Related to, but not entirely dependent on, the lifespan, is a dependent–independent continuum, the individual moving towards each end of the continuum dynamically depending upon the developmental stages of the lifespan, and immediate circumstances such as environment, state of health, etc. In living, the individual partakes of, or requires help with, four groups of activities, all of which are interrelated, and are only divided into discrete entities for the purpose of analysis:

activities of living
preventing activities
comforting activities
seeking activities

From these concepts, a model of living can be constructed (Table 1).

Roper, Logan and Tierney (1983) and Punton (1983) describe how the application of a nursing model in practice leads to greater patient involvement and to a broader, 'different' approach to the care of people. All of the models described in the literature view the recipient of nursing from a holistic perspective, see the goal of nursing as independence, or self-care for the patient, and define the knowledge base needed for nursing as a broad understanding of the physiology, psychology and sociology of human living (Pearson and Vaughan, 1986).

Such a concept of nursing is not, however, reflected in the reality of practice (Royal Commission on the National Health Service, 1979) or in the training curriculum for registered general nurses. The ideas inherent in such models may therefore be threatening to nurses who have been socialised

11

Table 1.1 Model of Living
(after Roper, Logan and Tierney (1980)).
Although all four groups of activities are so interrelated that in reality they cannot be seen to be separate, it is suggested by Roper, Logan and Tierney (1980) that discussion of them separately clarifies the nature of nursing.

Activities of living preventing comforting seeking	Conception ——lifespan——▶ Death Totally dependent ◀——continuum——▶ Totally independent
Maintaining a safe environment	_____
Communicating	_____
Breathing	_____
Eating and drinking	_____
Eliminating	_____
Personal cleansing and dressing	_____
Controlling body temperature	_____
Mobilising	_____
Working and playing	_____
Expressing sexuality	_____
Sleeping	_____
Dying	_____

into valuing highly the ideologies previously taught during training (Pearson and Vaughan, 1984b). Alternatives to the medical model are also fiercely criticised by doctors (Orem, 1980) because they suggest that the discipline of medicine is not necessarily the only, or even the most important, contributor to health care, so the supremacy of doctors must be questioned.

The nurse/patient relationship

The changes promoted by nursing leaders include advocating closeness between nurse and patient, the idea of partnership (Pearson, 1983; Punton, 1983), and the development of empathy in nursing. Such a change topples the current norms of practice which see the nurse as one who 'plies a trade' and has an air of professional detachment; it emphasises the patient's unique abilities and desires, and sees the role of the nurse as one of complementing these (Capra, 1983), through developing empathic ability.

Empathy is defined by La Monica (1977) as 'A word which

we use when one individual is hearing or understanding another. Empathy involves crawling inside of another person's skin and seeing the world through his eyes . . . Empathy involves experiencing another person's world as if you were he.' They assert that empathy is the primary ingredient in any helping relationship, a view with which Carkhuff (1969) agrees. Murray (1976) and Roper, Logan and Tierney (1980) argue for empathy training to be included in basic nurse education.

Rogers (1951) comments on the acquisition of empathic ability. He says that in any helping relationship, the helper must as far as he/she is able assume the internal frame of reference of he who is to be helped; perceive the world as he does; and communicate this empathic understanding, creating a non-threatening, accepting atmosphere, so the relationship can grow and be used in a helpful and constructive way. Alfano (1971) agrees with this thesis, and reports on the adoption of her concept of 'healing nursing' in a study involving a nursing unit in New York. The concept is based on the development of a close relationship between the nurse and patient, using this closeness to therapeutic effect. The results of the study show significant improvements in patient outcomes when compared with traditional practice in a variety of other settings. Rogers (1951) says that it is difficult to describe how warmth and empathy are communicated, and that it is essentially tremendously varied from one person to another. The ability to empathise is therefore, he argues, acquired in a different way by each individual, but has to grow from experience in interacting with others.

Nurses at present appear to maintain a distant, impersonal position, surrounding themselves (alongside other health workers) with an 'aura of mystery' (Friedson, 1970). They utilise the depersonalisation opportunities offered by the occupational structure (Menzies, 1960) and develop further aids to effect this distancing between nurse and patient, for example the widespread, unnecessary use of face masks (Roth, 1957). The 'new' practice orientation demands a nurse/patient relationship involving a nurse who is self-aware, able to cope with self-disclosure and with highly developed interpersonal relationship skills (Jourard, 1971; Argyle, 1972; Murray, 1976; Sundeen *et al.*, 1976; Schweer, 1972; McFarlane and Castledine, 1982).

Comparing the current norms of nursing practice, as evidenced by the literature with the 'new' norms being advocated by the nursing establishment, presents an overwhelming discrepancy between the two. Such a discrepancy suggests that if the new ideas are to become a part of reality, major, radical change will be necessary.

A rational, systematic approach to nursing

The nursing process is a method of individually planning and delivering nursing care, and has been one of the major innovations which clinical nurses have been exhorted to adopt.

Elhart *et al.* (1978) define the nursing process as 'the framework through which the nurse functions to meet specific responses in the provision of patient care'. Many authors base the process on the scientific problem-solving process (Hunt and Marks-Maran, 1979; McFarlane and Castledine, 1982), which has been adapted to fit the activities of a number of occupations. De Cecco (1974), for example, in describing a teaching model compares it, and most other teaching models, with the problem-solving process. Larkin and Backer (1977) suggest that without the ability to use problem-solving skills, nurses are 'forced to function by rote depending on memorised facts, and knowledge may be obsolete soon after a nurse graduates'. Johnson and Davis (1975) also see the skills involved in the nursing process as the same as those in problem-solving, which they see as 'the key technique in the nursing process'. Sundeen *et al.* (1976) however, differentiate between the problem-solving process and the nursing process: 'the problem-solving process is the development of new knowledge. The purpose of the nursing process is to maximise a client's positive interaction with his environment, his level of wellness and his degree of self-actualisation.'

Campbell (1978) sees the use of nursing process as 'the basis for professional practice which is flexible enough to serve as a skeleton for most nursing functions'.

The framework of a process gives logical steps through which to move, and different writers on the nursing process propose various components. Beland (1970) describes a ten-step process, with a number of substeps:

1. Observe
2. Measure and quantify

3. Communicate
4. Classify data, organise facts into related groups
5. Predict
6. Infer
7. Formulate hypotheses
8. Develop a plan of care
   a. State the patient's nursing needs and translate them into objectives of care
   b. Establish priorities
   c. Consider possible approaches
   d. Select appropriate nursing methods
   e. Make an appropriate plan
   f. Coordinate the plan with those of other patients in the group
   g. Coordinate and integrate all activities entering into the overall plan of therapy
   h. Anticipate future needs
9. Carry out the plan
   a. Inform the patient of the plan's details
   b. Carry out the plan
10. Evaluate.

Campbell (1978) lists six steps, Orem (1971) three, and Sundeen *et al.* (1976) five. Although Beland's ten-step process may be very comprehensive, its lengthiness makes it unpopular with nurses.

Roper, Logan and Tierney (1980, 1981, 1983) and Pearson and Vaughan (1984b) suggest the same four-step approach to the nursing process, summarising those of other writers:

1. Assessment
2. Planning
3. Implementation
4. Evaluation

Assessment

Assessment includes data collection, and identification of patient problems. Yura and Walsh (1973) describe the nursing assessment as the 'continuous systematic, critical, orderly, and precise method of collecting, validating, analysing and interpreting information about the physical, psychological and social

15

needs of a patient; the nature of his self-care deficits; and other factors influencing his condition and care'.

Gathering information is seen as the initial activity of assessment by Lewis (1968) who adds that a major part of this is in 'the interaction between the nurse and the person, which occurs when there is a meeting of meaning between them'. In order for data collected to be organised, assessment forms or frameworks are advocated by most writers. Murray (1976) says that 'a format that is systematic and efficient will be useful for obtaining the greatest amount of information in the shortest time'. More importantly, a predetermined framework is said to help in ensuring that all possible patient needs are considered, and none forgotten.

Yura and Walsh (1973) use the hierarchy of needs developed by Maslow as an assessment framework; Abdullah and Levine (1965) use a typology of 21 nursing problems they have developed; Marriner (1975) uses an acronym which acts as an *aide-mémoire* for body functions; Pearson and Vaughan (1984b) argue strongly that the basis for assessment should be a well-developed nursing model and Roper, Logan and Tierney (1981, 1983), Mayers (1972), Roy (1980) and others all present assessment formats based on nursing models. When data is collected, patient problems are identified, with close involve-ment of the patient (Tierney, 1984). Campbell (1978) says that 'for years, nurses have been using medical diseases as the basis for nursing care. But today, we are developing our own list of patient problems, which are not diseases, in an effort to establish a more precise nursing profession.'

Some authors use the identified problems to formulate a 'nursing diagnosis'. Marriner (1979) defines this as 'a statement or conclusion based on scientific principles and indicating the patient's need for nursing care'. When problems are identified a pattern emerges and the recognition of this pattern leads to a nursing diagnosis. It establishes a point of departure and basis for nursing care, and Murray (1976) says that the assessment step leads to a 'precise, concise and highly personalised statement of a nursing diagnosis which will begin the develop-ment of a nursing care plan'.

Planning

Written, explicit nursing care planning is the next process step. Stevens (1972) asserts that 'so many credible reasons can be given for the use of the nursing care plan, that the failure to write plans is puzzling'. She lists a number of reasons for written plans:

1. Nursing must be willing to identify its own content above and beyond the carrying out of medical orders.
2. Both consensus of nursing approach and continuity, with shift changes, etc. require a written plan of care.
3. Patient involvement with his own care demands that the plan be made explicit.
4. Writing a plan helps the nurse to clarify and solidify her goals.

Setting goals is seen as an integral and important component of care planning by Marriner (1979), Elhart *et al.* (1978), Mayers (1972), Bond (1984).

Implementation

Implementation is carrying out the plan, and includes consideration of the method of organising care.

Evaluation

Evaluation is regarded as a crucial, but often forgotten part of nursing. Elhart *et al.* (1978) say that 'whatever the tentative solution or nursing care plan, the process is not complete without arriving at some sort of judgement as to whether the problem has been resolved, unresolved, or created new problems'. They go on to say that evaluation must be continuous and both formal and informal. Mayers (1972) suggests that evaluation has been ignored in all health care occupations until recently because 'the mystique associated with all of the healing arts intimidated patients and professionals alike'. She deems it essential that 'all expected outcomes be evaluated in terms of the goals originally established'.

THE WAY AHEAD

The trend in nursing, then, is to encourage practitioners to base their practice on a model devised for nursing, through establishing a close therapeutic relationship between nurse and

17

patient, and by using a systematic, problem-solving approach to care.

Such a task is not appropriate for a subservient clinical nurse who is inferior to both medical staff and the hierarchy of nurses in management. It demands the development of a skilled practitioner who occupies a role which encompasses a degree of autonomy and clear accountability to the client. For this to happen, the status of the skilled nurse who remains at the side of the patient needs to be seen as equal to that of those nurses who pursue a career in management or teaching. At present this does not happen, and it is crucial that steps are taken to ensure that it does. Furthermore, the role of clinical nurses needs to be rethought. The role of a primary nurse, and the method of organising care based on the concept of primary nursing, seems to offer an excellent opportunity to both enhance the role of the direct care-giving nurse, and to create a structure through which the current trends can be put into practice.

REFERENCES

Abdullah, F.G. and Levine, E. (1965) *Better Patient Care through Nursing Research*. (Macmillan, New York).

Alfano, G.J. (1971) 'Healing or Caretaking — Which Will It Be?' *Nursing Clinics of North America*, 6, 273–280.

Argyle, M. (1972) *The Psychology of Interpersonal Behaviour*, 2nd edn. (Penguin Books, Harmondsworth).

Batchelor, I. (1980) *The Multi-disciplinary Clinical Team — A Working Paper*. (Kings Fund, London).

Beland, I.L. (1970) *Clinical Nursing: Pathophysiological and Psychosocial Approaches*. (Collier Macmillan, London).

Beyers, M. and Phillips, C. (1971) *Nursing Management for Patient Care*. (Little, Brown and Co., Boston).

Binnie, A. (1984) 'The Third Step of the Nursing Process — Implementation', in Bower, F.L. (ed.) *The Process of Planning Nursing Care*. (C.V. Mosby, St Louis).

Bond, S. (1984) 'The Second Step of the Nursing Process — Planning', in Bower, F.L. (1972) *The Process of Planning Nursing Care*. (C.V. Mosby, St Louis).

Bower, F.L. (1972) *The Process of Planning Nursing Care*. (C.V. Mosby, St Louis).

Byrne, M.L. and Thompson, L.F. (1978) *Key Concepts for the Study and Practice of Nursing*, 2nd edn. (C.V. Mosby, St Louis)

Campbell, C. (1978) *Nursing Diagnosis and Intervention in Nursing Practice*. (John Wiley and Sons, New York).

Capra, F. (1983) *The Turning Point. Science, Society and the Rising Culture*. (Fontana, London).

Carkhuff, Robert R. (1969) 'The Prediction of the Effects of Teacher-counselor Education: The Development of Communication and Discrimination Selection Indexes'. *Counselor Education Supervision*, 8, 4, 265–271.

Cartwright, A. (1964) *Human Relations and Hospital Care*. (Routledge and Kegan Paul, London).

Chapman, C. (1979) 'Sociological Theory Related to Nursing', in Colledge, M.M. and Jones, D. (eds), *Readings in Nursing*. (Churchill Livingstone, Edinburgh).

Davies, C. (1976) 'Experience of Dependency and Control in Work: the Case of Nurses'. *Journal of Advanced Nursing*, 1(4), 273–282.

Davies, C. (1977) 'Continuities in the Development of Hospital Nursing in Britain'. *Journal of Advanced Nursing*, 2(5), 479–493.

Davis, F. (1975) 'Professional Socialisation as Subjective Experience', in Cox, C. and Mead, A. (eds), *A Sociology of Medical Practice*. (Collier Macmillan, London).

De Cecco, J.D. (1974) *The Psychology of Learning and Instruction*. (Prentice-Hall, Englewood Cliffs, New Jersey).

Dickoff, J. and James, P. (1968) 'Researching Research's Role in Theory Development'. *Nursing Research*, 17, 204–206.

Duberley, J. (1977) 'How Will the Change Strike Me and You?'. *Nursing Times*, 73(45), 1736–1738.

Eardley, A. *et al.* (1975) 'Health Education by Chance'. *International Journal of Health Education*, 18(1), 19–25.

Elhart, D., Firsich, S.C., Gragg, S.H. and Rees, O.M. (1978) *Scientific Principles in Nursing*, 8th edn (C.V. Mosby, St Louis).

Friedson, E. (1970) *Professional Dominance. The Social Structure of Health Care*. (Aldine, Chicago).

Friedson, E. (1975) *The Profession of Medicine*. (Dodds, Mead and Co., New York).

Goffman, E. (1968) *Asylums*. (Penguin, Harmondsworth).

Gonzalez, F. (1981) 'How Should Nursing Be Managed Below the Level of Director of Nursing Services?' *Nursing Times*, 77, 14.

Hall, L.E. (1964) *Project report. The Solomon and Betty Loeb Center at Montefiore Hospital*. (The Centre, New York).

Henderson, V. (1966) *The Nature of Nursing*. (Collier Macmillan, London).

Hunt, J.M. and Marks-Maran, D.J. (1979) *Nursing Care Plans. The Nursing Process at Work*. (Heinemann Medical, London).

Johnson, M.M. and Davis, M.L.C. (1975) *Problem Solving in Nursing Practice*. (Wm C. Brown Co., Iowa).

Jourard, S. (1971) *The Transparent Self*. (D. Van Nostrand, New York).

Kratz, C. (1977) 'The Nursing Process'. *Nursing Times*, 73(23), 854–855.

La Monica, E.L. (1979) 'Empathy Training'. *Nursing Mirror*, 25 August, pp. 22–25.

Larkin, D.D. and Backer, B.A. (1977) *Problem-oriented Nursing Assessment*. (McGraw-Hill, New York).

Lewis, L. (1968) 'This I Believe . . . About the Nursing Process'.

Nursing Outlook, 16.5, 26–29.

MacGuire, J.M. (1980) *The Expanded Role of the Nurse*. (Kings Fund, London).

Marram, G. (1979) 'Perspectives in Nursing Management', in Marriner, A. (ed.), *Primary Nursing*, vol. 1, Ch. 8, pp. 84–92. (C.V. Mosby, St Louis).

Marriner, A. (1979) *The Nursing Process*. 2nd edn. (C.V. Mosby, St Louis).

Mayers, M.G. (1972) *A Systematic Approach to the Nursing Care Plan*. (Appleton-Century-Crofts, New York).

McFarlane, J.K. (1976) 'The Role of Research and the Development of Nursing Theory'. *Journal of Advanced Nursing*, 1, 443–451.

McFarlane, J. K. (1980) *The Multi-disciplinary team*. (Kings Fund, London).

McFarlane, J.K. and Castledine, G. (1982) *A Guide to the Practice of Nursing Using the Nursing Process*. (C.V. Mosby, London).

Menzies, I.E.P. (1960) 'Nurses Under Stress: A Social System Functioning as a Defence Against Anxiety'. *International Nursing Review*, 7.6, 9–16.

Metcalfe, C.A. (1982) 'Patient Allocation in a Maternity Ward: A Report of Some of the Findings', in Redfern, S.J., Sisson, A.R., Walker, J.F. and Walsh, P.A. (eds) *Issues in Nursing Research*. (Macmillan Press, London).

Meyer, V. (1981) *Unpublished dissertation* (University of Manchester, Department of Nursing).

Miller, E.J. and Gwynne, G.V. (1972) *A Life Apart*. (Tavistock, London).

Mitchell, J.R.A. (1984) 'Is nursing any business of doctors? A simple guide to the "nursing process" '. *British Medical Journal* 288, 216–219.

Murray, M. (1976) *Fundamentals of Nursing*. (Prentice-Hall, Englewood Cliffs, New Jersey).

Orem, D.E. (1971) *Nursing Concepts of Practice*. (McGraw-Hill, New York).

Orem, D. E. (1980) *Nursing: Concepts of Practice*, 2nd edn. (McGraw-Hill, New York).

Pavey, A.E. (1954) *The Story of the Growth of Nursing*, 3rd edn. (Faber, London).

Pearson, A. (1983) *The Clinical Nursing Unit*. (London, Heinemann Medical).

Pearson, A. and Vaughan, B.A. (1984a) 'Nursing Practice and the Nursing Process', in Open University Package P553 Modules 1 and 7, *A Systematic Approach to Nursing Care*. (Open University Press, Milton Keynes).

Pearson, A. and Vaughan, B.A. (1984b) 'Introducing Change into Nursing Practice', Open University Package P553 Modules 1 and 7, *A Systematic Approach to Nursing Care*. (Open University Press, Milton Keynes).

Pearson, A. and Vaughan, B.V. (1986) *Nursing Models for Practice*. (Heinemann, London).

Perrow, C. (1965) 'Hospitals: Technology, Structure and Goals', in March, J.G. (ed.) *Handbook of Organisations*. (Rand McNally, Chicago).

Punton, S. (1983) 'The Struggle for Independence'. *Nursing Times*, 2 March, 29–32.

Raphael, W. (1969) *Patients and their Hospitals*. (Kings Fund, London).

Reihl, J.P. and Roy, C. (1980) *Conceptual Models for Nursing Practice*. (Appleton-Century-Crofts, New York).

Reilly, D. (1975) 'Why a Conceptual Framework?' *Nursing Outlook*, 23, 9.

Reynolds, M. (1978) 'No News is Bad News: Patients' Views about Communication in Hospital'. *British Medical Journal*, 1, 1673–1676.

Rogers, C.R. (1951) *Client Centred Therapy*. (Houghton Mifflin, Boston).

Roper, N. (1976) *Clinical Experience in Nurse Education*. (Churchill Livingstone, Edinburgh).

Roper, N. (1979) 'Nursing based on a model of living', in Colledge, M.M. and Jones, D. (eds) *Readings in Nursing*. (Churchill Livingstone, Edinburgh).

Roper, N., Logan, W.W. and Tierney, A.J. (1980) *The Elements of Nursing*. (Churchill Livingstone, Edinburgh).

Roper, N., Logan, W.W. and Tierney, A.J. (1981) *Learning to Use the Process of Nursing*. (Churchill Livingstone, Edinburgh).

Roper, N., Logan, W.W. and Tierney, A.J. (1983). *Using a Model for Nursing*. (Churchill Livingstone, Edinburgh).

Roth, J.A. (1957) 'Ritual and Magic in the Control of Contagion'. *American Sociological Review*, 22, 310–314.

Rowden, R. (1984) 'Doctors Can Work with the Nursing Process: A Reply to Professor Mitchell'. *British Medical Journal*, 288, 219–221.

Royal College of Nursing Association of Nursing Practice (1980) *Clinical Career Structure*, unpublished.

Royal College of Nursing (1981) *A Structure for Nursing*. (RCN, London).

Royal Commission on the National Health Service (1979) Report. (HMSO, London).

Roy, C. (1980) 'The Roy Adaptation Model', in Reihl, J.P. and Roy, C. (eds) *Conceptual Models for Nursing Practice*. (Appleton-Century-Crofts, New York).

Schweer, J.E. (1972) *Creative Teaching in Clinical Nursing*. (C.V. Mosby, St Louis).

Smuts, J.C. (1926) *Holism and Evolution*. (Macmillan, New York).

Spelman, M.S., Ley, P. and Jones, C. (1966) 'How do we improve doctor–patient communications in our hospitals?' *World Hospitals*, 2, 126–134.

Stein, L. (1978) 'The Doctor–Nurse Game', in Dongwall, R. and McIntosh, J. (eds) *Readings in the Sociology of Nursing*, 107–117. (Churchill Livingstone, Edinburgh).

Stevens, B.J. (1972) 'Why Won't Nurses Write Nursing Care Plans?' *Journal of Nursing Administration*, 2, 6–7, 91–92.

Stockwell, F. (1972) *The Unpopular Patient*. (RCN, London).

Sundeen, S.J. *et al*. (1976) *Nurse–Client Interaction — Implementing the Nursing Process*. (C.V. Mosby, St Louis).

Szasz, T.S. and Hollender, M.H. (1975) 'Contribution to Philosophy of Medicine; Basic Models of Doctor–Patient Relationship. *AMA Archives of Internal Medicine*, 97, 585–592.

Tierney, A. (1984) 'The First Step of the Nursing Process — Assessment', in *A Systematic Approach to Nursing Care*. (Open University Press, Milton Keynes).

Tiffany, C.H. (1977) *Nursing, organizational structure and the real goals of hospitals; a correlational study*. Unpublished PhD study, Indiana University.

Travelbee, J. (1971) *Interpersonal Aspects of Nursing* (F.A. Davis, Philadelphia).

White, R. (1982) 'The Postwar Reconstruction of Nursing', in Redfern, S.J., Sisson, A.R., Walker, J.F. and Walsh, T.A. (eds) *Issues in Nursing Research*. (Macmillan Press, London).

Wiedenbach, E. (1964) *Clinical Nursing*. (Springer, New York).

Wilson, J. (1972) *Philosophy and Education Research*. (NFER, Windsor).

Yura, H. and Walsh, M.B. (1973) *The Nursing Process*. (Appleton-Century-Crofts, New York).

Zola, I.R. (1975) 'Medicine as an Institution of Social Control', in Cox, C. and Mead, A. (eds) *A Sociology of Medical Practice*, 170–185. (Collier Macmillan, London).

2

Primary Nursing

Alan Pearson

INTRODUCTION

Primary nursing is a simple return to the original way of delivering nursing, yet it could have a revolutionary effect on the services received by patients. It offers a chance to reaffirm the central importance in health care of the nurse who gives direct care, and the opportunity to make the 'trendy' factors in nursing a reality. Primary nursing is, however, simply a way of organising care, and this chapter outlines its underlying ideas.

ORGANISATION OF WORK

Nursing in all contexts is delivered alongside a multidisciplinary team. Any group activity needs organisation, which grows out of a need for cooperation and develops when an individual alone cannot achieve the desired goal by himself or herself. So direct care in a ward or community unit requires organisation and this day-to-day organisation is influenced by the wider organisation of the institution itself. The purpose of the hospital influences the organisation as a whole and the day-to-day organisation of care. The purpose of any hospital ward is caring for the patient either directly through actual patient care or indirectly through research and teaching, but the vested interests of professionalism often blur this purpose, and there is growing evidence in the United States that this overall purpose often takes second place to the aggrandisement of professions who seek more power. Other countries tend to follow the United States, so this is not an irrelevant issue. The factors that determine the quality of care a nurse is able to give include the ability of the nurse, the physical environment, the philosophy of the institution and the method of work organisation.

The welfare of patients cannot be controlled directly by their own actions when they are in hospital. It varies according to the doctors and nurses. In the relationships between caregivers and those who receive care there are few checks to prevent the abuse of power. Turner (1977) suggests that there are two possible attitudes that a power holder may have towards a dependant and these can be applied by the nurse to the patient. On one end of the continuum there is a dehumanising attitude that leads to ignoring or dismissal of the dependant's individuality. At the other extreme there is a humanitarian attitude, which preserves and cherishes individuality through attention to psychosocial needs.

This matches very much today's individualised focus of nursing. But using new documents or a nursing model rarely achieves such an effect. While using problem-solving, assessing, planning, implementing and evaluating may well lead to an intellectual pursuit of individuality, it is absolutely crucial that this is carried through by using a system of organising care that allows this to happen. Often this does not follow.

Traditionally, in the 1940s, 1950s and 1960s, nursing was organised fairly rigidly according to the assignment of tasks. This was the major form of organisation and although many dispute it, still exists widely in many hospitals throughout the world. So it is interesting to start our look at organising care with this method of assignment.

TASK ASSIGNMENT

Up until 1972 at least, 61 per cent of work in acute hospitals was still being allocated by tasks. In 1973 both Anderson (1973) and McLean (1973) confirmed that the completion of tasks and fulfilment of ward routine tended to provide more nurse satisfaction that patient-oriented goals. Other studies (for example Stockwell, 1972; and Hawthorn, 1974) report that when a nurse has completed her assigned task she tends to withdraw from the patient area until it is time to begin on the next one. Nurses feel guilty if they talk to patients and many do not feel that conversation constitutes work even when the ward is quiet. This was found by several studies to prevent care that would meet the individual needs of patients (Hayward 1975). Anderson (1973) also reported that 42 per cent of patients felt that not enough time was spent talking to them and answering their questions.

Task assignment is efficient, safe and cost-effective, and is said to have first been introduced because of the attachment of nursing in the past to the church and the armed services. Both of these traditions were strongly authoritarian and hierarchical and influenced the development of nursing long after it had become a purely secular occupation.

As nursing became more and more professional, an increasing distance developed between the qualified nurse and the fundamental task of nursing involving actual patient contact, for example, bathing, feeding etc. and these tasks were surrendered to unskilled or semiskilled assistants. The qualified nurses began to concentrate on technical procedures, many were brought up and socialised into valuing this and it became well established throughout this country.

It has also been said that this division of tasks occurred because of the adoption of an administrative rather than a professional authority model, while Menzies (1960) postulates that it was created from a social defence system that would reduce the anxiety created by close contact with the totality of individual patients and their illness. Whatever its origins, its efficiency, and its cheapness, task assignment clearly militates against individualising care, and a better deal for the patient will not become part of our reality. Although introduction of the nursing process can be criticised because it overconcentrates on the method of delivering nursing rather than on the nature of nursing itself, it has led to a desire to look at the content and nature of nursing. It has also led to interest in new approaches to organising care. Learning about the process has led to a shift in emphasis towards the importance of a nurse/patient relationship and a gradual acceptance that a professional model of practice rather than hierarchical administrative models would in the end improve the lot of the patient.

Marram (1979) says that good nursing includes:

● the unification of the patient's care to minimise fragmentation;
● the need to dismantle hierarchies so that well-qualified and skilled nurses can engage in direct patient care.

25

Such sentiments have, I think, come to be seen as desirable as a direct result of the use of the nursing process.

METHODS OF ORGANISING CARE

A number of methods of organising care have been explored and applied and it is useful to look at team nursing, day-to-day allocation, and progressive patient care before concentrating on primary nursing.

Team nursing

Team nursing, although introduced in North America almost 35 years ago (Leino, 1951; Lambertson, 1953) does not seem to have been developed much in the United Kingdom before the 1970s. In 1978 Marks Maran reported that the traditional concept of care was still that which revolves around routine and task allocation. Team nursing is a system of providing care by concentrating on the idea of good teamwork. It is, says Kron (1976), a philosophy rather than a method. It supports the achievement of goals through group action and is based on the belief that participative management increases job satisfaction and motivation.

Responsibility is decentralised and authority is delegated to a leader. The leader is a registered nurse who plans, gives and evaluates care, and communicates and delegates care to other members of the team who also participate in the process of nursing through the means of regular, daily team meetings. On the whole, however, experience suggests that it does not inevitably lead to individualisation of care. Its advantages are:

● the patient is more able to identify personnel who are responsible for his care;
● if the teams are constant, care becomes more continuous;
● it allows for the opportunity for the development of leadership in team members;
● it gives closer supervision to untrained and junior staff;
● it decentralises the authority of the ward sister.

Its major disadvantage, however, is that very often within the team task assignment still prevails.

Marram (1970) and Kramer (1971) criticise it as a method of care delivery and say that the demands on the team leader are too great. There is an overemphasis on supervision and task completion and assigning members to a group rarely leads to the making up of a team.

Progressive patient care (unit assignment)

Here teams are assigned patients on a geographical basis with varying degrees of dependency. In a system described by Sjoberg *et al.* (1971) care groups are identified — for example intensive care group, above average care, average care, minimal care — and patients are moved from area to area according to their nursing needs in an attempt to match the right mix of nursing staff. The ward structure is decentralised, and divided into care units for each of the four care levels. Each small care unit is complete in terms of equipment and facilities, and the nurse's station for each is situated close to the patients. Each day, the patient is reviewed, and placed in the care unit corresponding to the level in which he is classified. Within each care unit, nursing is patient-centred and the nursing team operates in the same way as that in team nursing.

Again, this has its serious critics. On the positive side it does make efficient use of personnel and equipment, and patients are put in the best place to receive appropriate care. However, its major disadvantages are that frequently patients become distressed at being moved often, continuity of care is very difficult and the nurse/patient relationship rarely develops well because of constant changes.

Day-to-day allocation of care

This has become the most widely used method second to task assignment. In this method, each day at the beginning of the shift a nurse is assigned to care for a group of patients. The nurse may be a student or qualified nurse, or a nursing auxiliary. For that shift the nurse gives total patient care. This has led to a more holistic approach, greater continuity for a shift, and in some places an individualised approach.

However, its major disadvantage is that the assignments change on a day-to-day basis. A nurse may look after a different group of patients for the five days she works in a week so therefore continuity is disrupted and the opportunity to develop a close nurse/patient relationship is less likely to occur.

PRIMARY NURSING EXPLORED

Primary nursing is, I believe, the most useful adjunct to identifying a model for nursing and operationally applying it through the use of the nursing process. It is a method of organising care that focuses on an individual nurse being responsible for a patient throughout his hospital stay. It is a method that has been used in community nursing since it began, and it is surprising that it has not been applied to institutional nursing. It is a development of the case method which was the practice norm until the 1930s according to Beyers and Phillips (1971), where one nurse performed all the nursing care for the patient.

The case method is not administratively or economically feasible for general adoption at the moment. Primary nursing is seen as a return to a case method with a primary nurse assuming responsibility for a caseload of patients throughout their hospital stay — or, in the case of district nursing, care by community services.

The primary nurse holds 24 hour, seven days a week responsibility for planning and administering care, although obviously only providing actual care during her hours on duty. When she is off duty, care is continued by an associate nurse. The associate nurse follows the care plan developed by the primary nurse, although Manthey et al. (1970) have suggested that the associate nurse may change parts of the care plan to reflect changes in the patient's condition. However, the primary nurse is responsible for any fundamental changes in the design of the plan.

Manthey (1973) and Manthey et al. (1970) describe the introduction of primary nursing in the United States in detail. A registered nurse on each ward was given primary responsibility for a group of patients numbering from three to six. The primary nurse assessed her patient on admission, prepared a care plan and was responsible for carrying out that plan and

28

evaluating it. When she was off duty, responsibility was delegated by her to an associate. The approach has been well accepted in the United States and is gaining popularity in this country.

It is ideally suited to a real implementation of holistic nursing using a systematic approach like that of the nursing process and can give the patient the opportunity to relate to his own nurse, who can then develop a close therapeutic relationship; together a partnership can be created so that individual needs can really be identified and an individual plan of action constructed by both nurse and patient together.

The greatest advantage of primary nursing is that the clinical nurse can begin to work in a professional way, and be accountable to an individual client for the care he needs. This, I believe, is the mark of individualising care.

Individualisation means, in effect, autonomy to the patient, but this cannot happen if the direct caregiver who is with him is powerless to allow him to carry out the decisions he makes. Autonomy for the nurse means autonomy for the patient.

Manthey, in discussing primary nursing, says:

> It is a system for delivering nursing care. That is all it is. It is not a solution to the problem of the difference between professional and technical levels of practice and preparation, it is not a solution to the issues created by the use of practical nurses, it will not solve staffing problems nor will it increase the workload. It will solve neither personnel management nor interpersonal relationship problems. It is innovation that works in the real world because that is the crucible in which it was originally developed and tested.

So primary nursing, like both the nursing process and the application of theory to practice, is not the panacea of all ills in isolation, but all these factors together can lead to a higher quality of nursing care.

THE OVERALL IMPLICATIONS OF PRIMARY NURSING

Most nurses are aware of the inadequacies of task allocation. The alternative methods of managing care focus on the patient and his needs, rather than on the needs of the care setting and institutional routines. The nursing process expands nursing and removes it from its current task orientation — which, with its associated division of labour and hierarchical supervision, is said to militate against personal accountability to the patient, and to encourage generalised accountability to the organisation.

Autonomy — the adjunct to accountability — is not an easily recognised norm in clinical practice. It is suggested that if accountability for our actions as practitioners is to become part of our reality as nurses, we need to stop hiding 'behind care given by routines, procedures, and policy statements' and end 'reflex practice'. Rye's (1982) frequently quoted comment that nurses must suffer from a permanent crick in the neck because they spend so much time looking upwards in the hierarchy, rings painfully true.

This hierarchical structure dissipates authority. Rye suggests that the degree of accountability is limited to the degree of authority vested in the individual nurse. If the nurse perceives herself as a professional person accountable to her patient, it should follow that she accepts the status with all the rights and responsibilities that go with it.

Thinking about how to give authority to the nursing caregiver has occupied much of our time in the Burford and Oxford Nursing Development Units. The question of how to organise care delivery in such a way as to give authority, and thus clear personal accountability, is crucial. Although we still have a long way to go, we are beginning to move towards an autonomous nursing role, in the context of a multidisciplinary clinical team where interdependence is important. Autonomy, in our view, is not incompatible with multidisciplinary teamwork.

How primary nursing works: a case history

Ted Hillman, age 74, is admitted to hospital. He has been complaining of shortness of breath and a tight feeling across his chest, and the doctor suspects a heart condition. The purpose of the admission is to carry out a series of tests to establish a diagnosis, and to decide what to do about it.

Both Mrs Hillman and her husband are apprehensive as they walk into the hospital. Eventually, a middle-aged lady bustles up to them, smiles and says 'Hello, Mr Hillman, I'm Brenda

Beard, and I am your nurse.' For the next 20 minutes or so Brenda and the Hillmans talk together, and Brenda begins to ease their apprehension. She has already talked with the doctor (he knows Brenda is to be Ted's nurse), she is familiar with Ted's condition, and knows what tests are planned. Now she wants to find out more about Ted.

She talks to him about his physical complaints. She asks about his daily routine: What are his daily activities? What kinds of food does he like? When, and for how long, does he sleep? Has he been in hospital before? There are questions for Mrs Hillman too. How will she get to the hospital? Will the rest of the family be visiting? Brenda encourages the Hillmans to ask questions too. They are concerned about these tests: What are they? Will they hurt? How will the results help the doctor in deciding what should be done? Brenda answers each question, and goes on to explain how she, together with Ted, will write a plan of care, which Ted can show to his wife and discuss if he wishes. She also carefully explains that she will be responsible for planning *all* Ted's nursing care throughout his stay, and for coordinating the care given by other members of the team. As she leaves the room, Brenda gives Mrs Hillman a card with the hospital telephone number, and her name on it, so that Mrs Hillman can ring and ask for her if she wants to make enquiries about Ted.

After Brenda has gone, Mrs Hillman helps her husband to unpack and settle in. They are both a bit more at ease now, and reassured that Brenda will be a big help to them in the days to come.

The interview has done even more than help. It has made Brenda understand that Ted is a person as well as a patient, and it has begun to establish the relationship Brenda and Ted need to carry through the nursing process. This is crucial because starting from the moment of his admission, the round-the-clock nursing Ted will receive is Brenda's responsibility. As a primary nurse she will give the care when she is on duty, and will be accountable for the care given by a colleague when she is off duty.

Accountability is retained for the 24 hours and the nurse does not hand it over at the end of the shift. Such a system lends itself to accountability for clinical care, and generalised accountability is replaced with personal accountability. Since Brenda is given full responsibility for the patient's nursing care, he has a

31

large investment of her care and interest. Her performance becomes measurable, and her competence is on the line. Outcomes of her care can be evaluated and accountability is fixed.

Fundamental changes

Introducing primary nursing on a wide scale in Britain requires a number of fundamental changes in nursing. Hegyvary and Haussman (1976) give the following key implications of primary nursing:

● If the care givers are to be autonomous and accountable they must be qualified nurses. Primary nursing thus demands a professional service, where direct care is given by registered nurses — a possibility advocated by the Royal College of Nursing, but which still seems to be a long way off.
●The role of nurse managers and ward sisters needs to be rethought. Full accountability can only be achieved if the caregivers have a degree of self-governance, similar to other professional groups. Each primary nurse needs considerable freedom in designing approaches to care, and the line management of a hierarchy is often incompatible with this professional autonomy. So the hierarchy needs flattening, an original aim of NHS reorganisation (which is not being achieved in some areas).
● Finally, creative efforts to establish patterns of peer review and quality assurance programmes need to be made.

In the Burford and Oxford Nursing Development Units we are playing around with these ideas. Decisions about general policies which must be made for the benefit of the teamwork are made by the primary nurses as a group. The supervisory role has changed to become one of consultant and enabler. Qualpacs (Wainwright and Burnip, 1983) and nursing audit are being developed as tools for peer review and form the basis of peer discussions. Although we still have far to go, and our position is somewhat immature, a climate of creativity and evidence of a desire for autonomy and accountability glimmer through.

It is interesting that the 'centres of excellence' set up at

Chicago and Rochester in the United States, the professorial nursing unit at Manchester, and a number of progressive psychiatric units in this country have all chosen primary nursing (or the keyworker system) as an organisational framework Experience in all these units suggests that the approach is practical and meaningful to nurses; accountability is made explicit, and this leads to greater satisfaction for patients and nurses alike.

The emphasis on the one-to-one client-professional relationship is similar to that of doctors, and thus the facilitation of a professional model of practice with its associated autonomy and accountability in our view makes primary nursing the method of choice in organising care.

BURFORD AND OXFORD NURSING DEVELOPMENT UNITS

Both units are part of the British National Health Service, but have been additionally financed by major grants from the Sainsbury family trusts. The philosophy of nursing is the same in both units and thus the style of nursing and the staffing structure are the same. Staff are therefore able to interchange when necessary. The two units themselves are, however, different in their location, facilities and service.

Burford Nursing Development Unit (BNDU)

This is a small 12-bed unit which serves a well-defined rural population. In addition to the inpatient facilities, there is also a 50-place day unit, an outpatients department, a 24 hour casualty department, a district nursing service and a health visiting service. In essence, the BNDU is a community unit, which is nursing-oriented but also closely linked with primary medical and social services. Medical input to the unit comes from local family doctors. Social work, physiotherapy and occupational therapy are part of the unit. Originally a cottage hospital established in the 19th century, the Burford unit has longstanding traditions, and the current approach to nursing constitutes a major change to many of the health workers and clients who use the unit.

Oxford Nursing Development Unit (ONDU)

This was established in 1985, and recruited staff who were aware of the philosophy, and who therefore wished to adopt it. It is a 16-bed ward within a general hospital. Medical input comes from a part-time medical officer employed by the unit, and advice is given at a weekly team meeting by the medical adviser, who is an NHS consultant. Physiotherapy, occupational therapy and social work are provided by departments which serve the rest of the hospital.

REORGANISING MANAGEMENT TO FACILITATE PRIMARY NURSING

The hierarchical structure of the unit has been dismantled and a horizontal structure has replaced it (Figure 2.1). The key person for the patient is the primary nurse; the consultation link and other team members serve to support the primary nurse. The beliefs on which practice is based have been made explicit, and there are in-depth discussions on the attitudes of nurses and the rest of the team to age, illness and professional power. Nurses are given the opportunity to extend their knowledge; the primary nurse is encouraged and has permission to teach others, use research findings, decide on the management of care and conduct research if needed. The approach to care follows the problem-solving method.

The primary nurse is personally accountable to the patient, and is monitored by her primary nurse colleagues through peer reviews based on quality assurance exercises conducted by clinical peers from outside the unit. Nursing is seen as the major therapy, all care being given by qualified nurses. Nursing beds, funded by a charitable body, are currently being used for patients who are admitted in a biological crisis to an acute hospital. This is part of a study to measure the effect of nurses practising in a unit which focuses on nursing as an activity which is therapeutic in itself, as well as being complementary to medicine.

The role of the head of the unit has developed into one which is mainly consultation and the unification of the four branches of nursing: research, teaching, practice and management of care. As far as unification of those four aspects of nursing is

Figure 2.1 The Horizontal Structure Has Replaced the Old Hierarchical Structure (Source: Pearson, 1984).

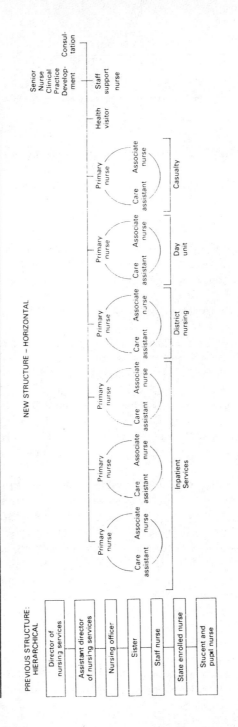

concerned, the role revolves around practising in the hospital, teaching nurses, researching and supervising the nurses who are carrying out research and managing care in the unit.

Consultation

Consultation, along this horizontal structure and throughout the district, makes up the other half of the job, and has been described as consisting of the following components.

- A process involving continual progression through a number of stages from the beginning to a defined end.
- A data-gathering enterprise in which needs are identified and actions are taken, based on the most current appraisal of data and feedback.
- A vehicle for assistance in the various forms of insight, understanding, knowledge and skill transfer, and for changing systems.
- An interpersonal relationship between two or more people or systems, each assuming specific roles and each affecting and being affected by the other.
- A voluntary arrangement in which the consultant has no administrative responsibility for the consultee or for implementing recommendations, and the consultee has the freedom to accept, modify or reject the consultant's contributions (summarised from Archer, Kelly and Bisch, 1984).

Within the nursing development units, though, the head is charged with administrative responsibility, and overall day-to-day management of the unit is delegated to a staff support nurse in each section — that is, one at Oxford and one at Burford. The responsibility of the head is to be available for consultation to unit nurses, when these five components can be applied. Most consultations are about patient care, nursing problems, management of care and the use of resources. Primary nurses have the freedom to accept, modify or reject contributions, given that they are accountable for the outcomes of care.

Many nurses are capable of working autonomously and are competent at reviewing each other's work effectively. From the early results of the nursing beds project, patient outcomes from the nursing unit compare favourably with those of patients in acute units, or similar community hospitals, which have not pursued developing nursing yet. We have also learned that primary nurses enjoy greater job satisfaction.

Clinical nurses need permission from nursing management to be creative and to take risks. They must also have the resources and opportunity to introduce a fairly heavy staff development programme to increase knowledge and skill bases and to provide experiential workshops to help nurses examine their attitudes. Support from other members of the multidisciplinary team, such as doctors, occupational therapists, physiotherapists and social workers, is required. Clinical nurses also need stamina, a thick skin and peer support.

There have been no increased financial costs; in fact, the changes have led to more cost effective use of the unit.

Hall (1964) said: 'The medical aspect of nursing has grown and grown so that something had to go. What went was the nurturing process which now the nurse, in turn, delegated to less well-prepared persons.' She regards nurturing as 'first-class nursing' and the carrying out of medically related tasks as 'second-class doctoring'. Though I cannot entirely agree, I think 'first class nursing' must emphasise nurturing, and that advanced nursing practice must stem from that.

Our experience suggests that we still have far to go, but we are more convinced that advanced practice must be developed at the primary nurse level. We have to go on making mistakes and taking risks if this is to happen.

NURSING PRACTICE WITHIN THE UNITS

Nursing care for an individual patient is the responsibility of his/her own primary nurse. In the Oxford unit, primary nurses are expected to teach, research and manage the unit on a day-to-day basis, and because of this increased responsibility and autonomy are known as nurse/practitioners. In the Burford unit, primary nurses are supported by a nurse practitioner who coordinates the work of the various departments; they are known simply as primary nurses. The only other worker in contact with patients is the care assistant, who both assists nurses and carries out all domestic work. Nursing auxiliaries and domestic assistants are not employed in the units.

Nursing practice is firmly based on a belief in primary nursing delivered through an all-registered nurse team:

- the need for a high level of support of non-nursing staff who are accountable to nursing;
- that nursing in itself is a therapy;
- the need for a close therapeutic relationship between nurse and patient;
- the power of touch in healing patients.

The following chapters expose these beliefs in detail, and describe how they are applied in practice. For reasons of clarity the primary nurse is referred to as 'nurse practitioner' throughout the book.

REFERENCES

Anderson, E.R. (1973) *The Role of the Nurse.* (RCN, London).

Archer, S.E., Kelly, C.D. and Bisch, S.A. (1984) *Implementating Change in Communities: A Collaborative Process.* (C.V. Mosby, St Louis).

Beyers, M. and Phillips, C. (1971) *Nursing Management for Patient Care.* (Little, Brown, Boston).

Hall, L. (1964) Project Report: The Solomon and Betty Loels Center at Montefiore Hospital, New York. Loels Center for Nursing.

Hawthorn, P. (1974) *Nurse I Want My Mummy.* (RCN, London).

Hayward, J. (1975) *Information, a Prescription against Pain,* RCN Research Series. (RCN, London).

Hegyvary, S.T. and Haussman, R.K.D. (1976) 'Monitoring Nursing Care Quality'. *Journal of Nursing Administration,* 6, 9.

Kramer (1974) *Reality Shock,* Mosby, St Louis).

Kron, T. (1976) *The Management of Patient Care.* (W.B. Saunders, Philadelphia).

Lambertson, E.C. (1953) *Nursing Team Organisation and Functioning.* (Columbia University Press, New York).

Leino, A. (1951) 'Organizing the Nursing Team'. *American Journal of Nursing,* 151, 665–667.

Manthey, M., Ciske, K., Robertson, P. *et al.* (1970) 'Primary Nursing'. *Nursing Forum* 9(1), 64–83.

Manthey, M. (1973) 'Primary Nursing is Alive and Well in Hospital'. *Nursing Forum,* 9(1), 65.

Marks-Maran, D. (1978) 'Patient Allocation v. Task Allocation in Relation to the Nursing'. *Nursing Times,* 74(10), 413–416.

Marram, G.D. (1970) 'Incorporating Supervised Supervision in the Graduate Curriculum'. *Nursing Outlook* 18(9), 46–47.

Marram, G.D. (1979) 'Perspectives in Nursing Management', in Marriner, A. (ed.) *Primary Nursing,* vol. 1, Chapter 8, 84–92.

(C.V. Mosby, St Louis).

McLean, J.P. 'Nursing Care Study: Bilateral Nephrectomy'. *Nursing Mirror*, 136(10), 31–34.

Menzies, I.E.P. (1960) 'Nurses Under Stress: A Social System Functioning as a Defence Against Anxiety'. *International Nursing Review*, 1 (6), 9–16.

Pearson, A. (1974) 'Quality Patient Care Scale', in Wessex Regional Health Authority *Report on Proceedings of Senior Staff Seminar on Quality Assurance*, Wessex.

Sjoberg, K. *et al.* (1971) 'Unit Assignment: A Patient Centred System'. *Nursing Clinics of North America*, 6, 2.

Stockwell, F. (1972) *The Unpopular Patient*. (RCN, London).

Turner, V. (1977) 'How the Nurse Can Help Preserve a Patient's Individuality'. *Nursing Mirror*, 144(3), 50–54.

Wainwright, P. and Burnip, S. (1983) 'Qualpacs at Burford', *Nursing Times*, 79(5), 36–38.

3

Primary Nursing in Practice

Richard McMahon

INTRODUCTION

> If it is virtually impossible for experienced nurses to relate nursing theory to everyday practice, then something is very wrong with either theory or practice.
>
> Miller 1985, p. 417.

The purpose of this chapter is to demonstrate that the concepts and theories involved in primary nursing can be successfully applied to practice by describing how these have been implemented in the nursing development units (NDUs). The roles of the units' staff differ markedly from those found on traditional wards, but paramedical services are provided by workers who also have responsibilities to other areas. In order to ensure a practical description of this implementation of primary nursing, emphasis is placed on the roles and interactions between the unit-based and non-unit-based staff. This somewhat structural account of the unit is followed by a description of the formal meetings that provide communication amongst the unit-based staff.

There is more involved in the implementation of primary nursing than simply changing the organisation of the nurses and ancillary workers. The concept of therapeutic care, involving nurse–patient partnership and patient autonomy is central to primary nursing and therefore to the practice of nursing in the unit. This is manifested in practices such as a non-directive approach to nursing, and the nurses on the unit not wearing uniforms. So while this chapter examines structural aspects of primary nursing, a discussion of the functional features of nurs-

Figure 3.1 The Linear Structure of Primary Nursing (adapted from Pearson, 1984).

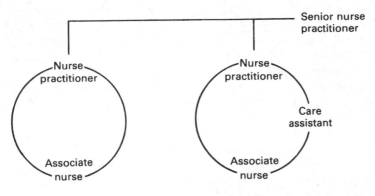

ing practice is provided by Plaxy-Anita Muetzel in Chapter 5.

Burford nursing development unit opened three nursing beds in 1983, and the Oxford nursing development unit, consisting of 16 nursing beds, opened in October 1985, accepting its first referrals in November. The purpose of both units was initially as a research project to show the effectiveness of a clinical nursing unit in terms of patient outcomes. The nature of a clinical nursing unit is described in detail in Chapter 4 by Steven Ersser, but simply the units accept patients whose greatest need is nursing, and who do not require specialist medical care. For the purposes of the research only three diagnostic groups are accepted, with patients being referred two or three days after their biological crisis. Currently, a lower age limit of 60 years is adhered to. At the conclusion of the research, diagnosis and age should no longer become criteria for referral.

Manthey (1980) suggests that one way of organising primary nursing is to have a number of primary nurses on a ward, each taking responsibility for a small number of patients. Thus when one of these nurses is on duty, she acts as a primary nurse for her own patients, and also as an associate nurse for her colleagues' patients on days off. However, in the NDUs primary nurses are responsible for eight patients each, and as there are always two nurses on duty they very rarely act as associate nurse for the other's patients. Consequently, the full-time associates only act as primary nurses when the nurse practitioner is on annual leave. All the nurses on the unit are registered nurses; the relationship between the nurse practitioner, associate nurses and unqualified care assistants is represented diagrammatically in Figure 3.1, in which either the nurse practitioner or an associate nurse is on duty caring for each group of eight patients, with the aid of the care assistants. This structure has significantly lower staffing costs than similar wards in the same hospital.

Before the roles of workers on the unit are discussed it should be emphasised that this work is descriptive of primary nursing as it has been implemented in *one* area. It is not intended as a 'blueprint' to be imposed elsewhere, instead it is meant as a catalyst to stimulate interest in primary nursing by showing that it does work in practice. Problems that have been encountered are included together with the steps taken to overcome them.

In the following analysis, unit-based staff are those who work exclusively on the Unit and are employed out of its budget. Non-unit-based staff are those health workers that have responsibility in a number of wards or areas, such as the physiotherapist, and who consequently are budgeted separately.

NURSE PRACTITIONERS (PRIMARY NURSES)

The primary nurses have the official title of nurse practitioners, to indicate that their role includes lecturing and research responsibilities as well as clinical practice, and that they are autonomous practitioners of nursing. However, these extra duties take up less than 10 per cent of the nurse practitioners' time, their major role being that of a primary nurse. As a manager the nurse practitioner also has responsibility for supervising the work of the care assistants, coordinators and activities' organiser.

The nurse practitioner movement originated in Colorado in 1965, at a time when the profession in America was 'clamouring for nurses to become increasingly clinical . . . orientated toward research in patient care, health based, autonomous, accountable and advanced in knowledge and skills' (Loretta Ford in Silver *et al*, 1985).

In that first programme involving nurse practitioners, the aim was to improve the health care of children and their families in rural and urban areas, and to expand the nurse's role. Since then, nurse practitioners have spread into areas of practice involving many diagnoses, age groups and locations. In some cases nurse practitioners have extended their roles to include some of the tasks traditionally performed by junior house doctors; however that was not the objective of the movement. The expanded role envisaged from that original Colorado project was one of nurses who are experts in clinical nursing based on health and patient-centred care and who also teach and perform clinical research (Ford, 1979). It is these aims that form the basis for the role of nurse practitioner in the nursing development units.

Therefore, the nurse practitioner role is mainly one of an autonomous clinical nurse who is responsible for eight patients. Manthey (1970) suggests that several factors should affect the ratio of patients to primary nurses. These include: rate of patient turnover; amount of medical intervention required; the number of non-nursing personnel involved in supporting care; the health education requirements of the patients; and the effectiveness of the support services. Therefore, in the nursing development units where the minimum stay is one week, efficient support for the nurses is provided, and the amount of medical intervention is small, a high patient-to-primary nurse ratio is achieved.

Admission of patients

When a patient is admitted his nurse practitioner commences an assessment as soon as feasible, based on the framework provided by Roper, Tierney and Logan (1985). This assessment is not regarded as a singular event, rather an ongoing process that over a period of days provides a unique profile of the patient. From this data the nurse practitioner extracts two types of information. The first is details of the likes and dislikes of the patient and a plan of his usual routine. This knowledge allows the environment and care to be moulded around the usual practices of the patient in an attempt to reduce the stress of hospitalisation and perhaps aid rehabilitation. The flexibility in the ward environment is achieved by having no routines other than those of the patients. Waking and retiring, breakfast, bathing, exercising and taking medication can all be timed by the patient's home routine. Similarly, patients' usual practices in washing, dressing, interacting and fulfilling spiritual needs

43

can normally remain unchanged. It is only the limitations of the physical environment and the services from outside the ward, such as the central kitchen, that impose restrictions on the patient's day.

The second type of information extracted from the assessment is the identification with the patient of those of his problems that are amenable to nursing intervention. From this discussion with the patient and his family the nurse practitioner negotiates a proposed discharge date towards which the team work.

Care planning

The planning of care with the patient is almost exclusively the responsibility of the nurse practitioner. For each of the problems identified from assessment, achievable goals are negotiated with the patient, with the prescribed care required to achieve those outcomes. Much of the prescribed care involves teaching patients and their families about their disabilities and the ways that they may be overcome. Where appropriate the nurse includes a preventive health education programme in the care plan. This emphasis on teaching and working with patients and their families rather than 'doing for' them reflects Pembrey's belief that: '. . . we can derive professional nursing as a partnership with the individual, with the nurse working primarily as a teacher' (Pembrey, 1984).

When care is planned by an associate nurse in the nurse practitioner's absence, it is the prerogative of the nurse practitioner as the person accountable for patient care to change that plan on her return if she feels it is inappropriate. Where possible, the prescribed care should be based on nursing research, or have a recognisable derivation from another relevant discipline such as physiology or psychology.

Delivery and evaluation of care

The nurse practitioner as care planner is also the principal caregiver, enabling her to develop a close therapeutic relationship with the patient. When on duty the nurse practitioner is the only nurse caring for her patients, with various support staff to perform the non-nursing duties traditionally undertaken by nurses. The nurse practitioner becomes the centre of communication for her patients. By having specific assessments of problems and observable patient-centred goals, the nurse practitioner can evaluate the effectiveness and appropriateness of the nursing interventions prescribed.

Some aspects of the care given by the nurse practitioners may be considered extended practices. Nurses on the units perform venepuncture and record electrocardiographs. This has not arisen out of a strong desire to perform these tasks, but rather out of the unit's philosophy, suggesting that it would be inappropriate for outside technicians to be called in when a person the patient knows and trusts is capable of doing them. Furthermore, with the medical officers only working part-time, doctors would have to be called in order to perform these tasks at weekends or early in the morning if the nurses could not do them, causing delays for patients.

Discharge of patients

It has already been stated that at the initial assessment the nurse practitioner discusses discharge plans with the patient and his family. At this time the location and date of discharge expected by the patient, and the level of recovery required for him to leave hospital, is ascertained. Clearly during the admission either the date or place of discharge may be altered as the patient perceives his progress. The final decision to discharge a patient is the consensus opinion of the multidisciplinary clinical team. This decision is frequently made after a visit to the patient's home by the patient, his nurse practitioner and representatives of any other disciplines involved in his care, to observe how he will cope in his home environment.

Accountability

Patients are admitted to the units because their greatest need is for nursing, and that care is planned and implemented by the nurse practitioner. Therefore, the nurse practitioner may be asked to account to the patient and his family, her own profession or to other members of the team for the quality of the care that is given. When the nurse practitioner is not on duty she puts her trust for the care of her patients in the hands of her associate nurses to perform the care she has prescribed. In this way the nurse practitioner is still accountable for the planned care even when not on the premises. Should a care plan suddenly become inappropriate, then the associate nurse on duty is required to contact the nurse practitioner to inform her of the change in the patient's condition and to confirm changes in the care plan.

Bergman (1981) suggests that there are three preconditions for accountability. The first of these is *ability*. The nurse practitioner cannot be held accountable for her care unless she has the necessary knowledge, skills and values to act on specific issues. The second factor is *responsibility*. The nurse practitioner is responsible for the nursing care received by her patients; she cannot be considered responsible and therefore accountable for the professional decisions of her colleagues, for example, the medical staff. The final precondition identified by Bergman is *authority*. A nurse cannot accept accountability for the care of patients unless she is given the authority to make decisions that affect that care. Primary nursing clearly gives the authority to make decisions to the primary nurse, so in the nursing development units where the nurse is recognised as the key worker, the nurse practitioner is ultimately accountable for care.

ASSOCIATE NURSES

The role of associate nurse is fulfilled by registered nurses. When the nurse practitioner is off duty, her patients are cared for by one of her associate nurses. Maintenance of individualised care in a consistent manner is achieved in two ways. Firstly, the nurse practitioner gives a verbal handover to her associate in the presence of the patient. This consists of a brief update of any changes that have occurred since the associate was last on duty. The overlap between shifts is generally only 15 minutes so that only essential information is conveyed about each of the eight patients. The second and principal means of maintaining continuity is through the use of written care plans, which provide a precise guide for the associate nurse of the care required by her patients. From these two methods of communication the associate nurse fulfils her role of implementing prescribed care.

The associate nurses act as the eyes and ears of the nurse practitioners, and in this way fulfil the evaluation part of the nursing process. By careful observation, the associate nurse is able to compare the patient's behaviours and conditions with those described in the assessment, and those stated as expected outcomes in the goal statements. These observations are generally made on the review date stated on the care plan for each problem; however, if there is a significant change this may be recorded at any time. The evaluation made by the associates should be accurately documented in the progress notes.

The associate nurses on the unit are also expected to contribute to the patient's assessment if they make observations not already considered. For example, a night associate nurse is often in a better position to assess a patient's current sleeping difficulty than the nurse practitioner. Minor changes to care plans may be made independently by the associate nurse to keep the plans up to date until the nurse practitioner is again on duty. Major changes are only made in consultation with the nurse practitioner.

There is also a small management component to the associate nurse role comprising of supervision of the care assistants and coordinators, maintenance of the safety of all persons on the unit, and dealing with the property and valuables of the patients in a responsible manner.

SENIOR NURSE PRACTITIONER

Manthey (1973) describes the role of the senior nurse on a primary nursing unit as: '. . . the factor most critical to the success of primary nursing'. The senior nurse practitioner post comprises a number of factors. The first of these is as an adviser on clinical nursing. To fulfil this part of the role the senior nurse practitioner should be an experienced clinical nurse, who has been, or has a good understanding of acting as, a primary nurse. She may be approached by the nurse practitioners for advice, and acts as a facilitator for the nurse practitioners to increase their clinical knowledge by performing literature searches or encouraging their attendance on courses or conferences. The senior nurse practitioner still practices, by acting as an associate nurse during periods of absence by staff.

The second function of the senior nurse practitioner is to provide psychological support for staff. This advisory and counselling capacity is of particular use to new staff who are unused to the positions of primary or associate nurses having previously worked in the conventional hierarchical system. The support provided is not only available to the nurses, but to any member of the ward team.

The next, and potentially most time-consuming part of her role is as manager. This involves keeping a record of annual leave and sickness, ensuring that these duties are covered, dealing with staff time-sheets and the appointing of new staff. Accountability to the health authority for the control of the unit's budget is vested in the senior nurse practitioner. Should a member of staff require disciplining, the senior nurse practitioner is involved only at the invitation of one of the nurse practitioners. Also within the managerial component of this post is that all patients referred to the unit are visited, so that they can be screened for the correct age and diagnosis (whilst the research project is running) and it can be decided whether the patient's greatest need is nursing. This visit also provides an opportunity for the patient to meet someone from the unit who can give a full explanation of where he is being transferred and for what reason.

Finally, the senior nurse practitioner coordinates the educational and research programmes held on the unit. This involves the planning and teaching of courses appropriate for the different grades of staff on the unit, the majority of courses being available to only qualified nurses interested in clinical practice. Approval for use of the unit for research projects has to be obtained from the senior nurse practitioner, who also encourages research projects by the unit's nurses.

MEDICAL OFFICER

In the Oxford unit, a medical officer is employed by the unit, and is responsible for providing a non-specialist medical service to its patients. Employed on a part-time basis, the doctor visits four or more times a week to order investigations and to deal with the routine medical problems of hospitalised patients. When not on duty the doctor may be contacted at home for advice. Unless the unit's medical officer is present on the ward, should a patient suddenly become ill the conventional on-call medical staff for the hospital provide the necessary service, which in extreme cases may require the patient to be returned to the acute area. In the Burford unit, medical care is provided in the same way, but by the general practitioners. One of the major criteria for admission to the unit is that patients should not need specialist medical care that requires a daily visit by the doctor. This is not a decision that a nurse is professionally qualified to make, therefore the unit medical officer also visits all referrals prior to acceptance for transfer to judge whether the stated criteria are met.

CARE ASSISTANTS

Staffing in the nursing development units is designed to provide maximum support to the nurses, to allow them more time to be involved in patient care. One of the ways this is achieved is by providing staff to perform the non-nursing duties traditionally done by nurses. Care assistants have as their primary role assisting the nurses in patient care, and are responsible to them, but this should not be confused with the work done on the other wards by auxiliaries, who are often involved in such activities as washing or bathing patients. In the nursing development units helping a patient to bath is recognised as a nursing activity and is therefore performed by a nurse. However, the nurse can arrange the time for the bath with the patient, and a care assistant then runs the bath and prepares the bathroom in advance with the patient's toiletries. Care assistants assist the nurses with lifting and other care requiring two persons. They also perform such tasks as bedmaking and urine testing that do not require specialist training. A series of prepared trays, set up for activities such as observing the patient's vital signs or examining and evacuating his/her rectum, are available for the care assistant to bring to the bedside for the nurse.

When not assisting the nurses care assistants carry total responsibility for keeping the ward clean and serving the meals. Each morning and evening they must complete a checklist of tasks that should have been performed on that shift so that anything there has not been time to complete can be made a priority for the next shift. At Oxford nursing development unit the cleaning of the floors is performed by private contractors, but care assistants at Burford nursing development unit also maintain the floors.

WARD COORDINATORS

The role of the ward coordinators on the unit is to take many of the administrative tasks from the nurses, and also to act as a filter for incoming information into the unit. They also provide a secretarial and data-processing service, which includes typing and keeping a filing system, and feeding research data into the computer: they are accountable to the nurse practitioners.

Administrative work — such as ordering, making appointments, arranging repairs to equipment, or writing out the basic duty rota — does not require the specialist skills of a nurse (although a nurse may be consulted), and may be successfully carried out by the ward coordinators. Also, as a huge amount of information is received by the unit each day it is the responsibility of the ward coordinators to deal with simple enquiries and circulars, while any information requiring the attention of a nurse is passed on to the appropriate person.

The coordination of communications is achieved in several ways.

1. The ward coordinators' office is at the entry to the ward so that visitors to the unit from both inside and outside the hospital have easily accessible contact with the ward. The ward coordinators deal with simple enquiries and direct visitors to the appropriate bed or area of the ward. Where the attention of a nurse is required the ward coordinator contacts the appropriate primary or associate nurse on duty by using a two-way radio carried by each nurse. This form of communication is necessary because the nurses spend most of their time in patient areas making locating one particular nurse in the various siderooms, toilets and bathrooms particularly time-consuming. By using the radio the nurse can be made aware that there is a visitor requiring her attention and she may respond by instructing the ward coordinator, for example, to ask the visitor to take a seat and tell him that the nurse will be down in five minutes. This system enables the nurse to complete the care she was giving while at the same time dealing promptly with visitors.

2. All incoming mail comes to the ward coordinators' office for sorting and redistribution.
3. All telephone calls are directed to the ward coordinators' desk, with two-way radios enabling the ward coordinator to tell the individual nurse where there is a call about one of her patients, and also ascertain whether or not the call will be taken in the office or at the nurses' station.

By coordinating the simple administrative and communication activities on the ward on a seven-day-a-week basis, the ward coordinators provide more time for the nurses to care for their patients. The importance of the ward coordinators as a 'filter' for incoming information is considered again on p. 55.

ACTIVITIES ORGANISER

A correlation between recreational activities throughout life and successful ageing was demonstrated in 1974 by DeCarlo. However, the provision of intelligent stimulating recreation for patients in hospital has rarely been a priority. An activities organiser provides activities and entertainments for patients on three afternoons a week in the nursing development units. These entertainments take such forms as dance, drama, music, or slide shows, which may be performed either by amateur or professional performers giving their services free. Many of these activities are likely to appeal to a large proportion of patients; however, when each patient is admitted the activities organiser tries to get to know him or her, and establish any likes and dislikes. This can lead to individualised activities such as playing cards or doing crosswords, or taking a group of patients to a cafe or a public house.

The extension of these entertainments into activities of a more interactive nature is encouraged by the ward staff. For example, an art project was included in the activities, involving the taking and developing of photographs by patients and staff as well as the photographer. Other activities include a reminiscence group, and bringing patients' pets into the ward.

NON-UNIT-BASED STAFF

The unit calls on a number of staff that have responsibility to a number of wards and who are not employed out of the unit's budget.

Medical consultant

Oxford nursing development unit is primarily for patients requiring intensive nursing care, resulting in an altered role for the medical consultant from that provided by the traditional model. In general, the consultant visits the unit once a week to attend the multidisciplinary review, in which he provides expert medical knowledge and advice to the team and in particular to the unit's medical officer. Clearly it is inappropriate for him to perform a ward round, so should the medical officer or nurse practitioner request that he examines a patient, this is performed before or after the review in the presence of the nurse practitioner. At Burford nursing development unit, all medical input comes from patients' own general practitioners.

Paramedical staff

These include: dietician, occupational therapist, physiotherapist, social worker, and speech therapist.

Each one is acknowledged as being a professional with expert knowledge. Nearly all the paramedical therapies are involved in teaching the patient and his family new knowledge or skills. However, none of these paramedical staff provides a 24 hour availability to the patient. In our nursing development units the nurse practioner is the member of the team who probably knows the patient best, and the associate nurses provide continuity of care in her absence. When this is considered with the 24 hour care provided by the nurses it seems reasonable that the nurse should be familiar with the basic therapies and services of her paramedical colleagues, so that these can be delivered or reinforced by staff with whom the patient is familiar when the specialist in that field is off the unit. To a certain extent this modifies the role of the paramedical staff to one of consultancy, in which they bring specialist expertise to the units.

Some therapists may find the role of 'consultant' a difficult one to accept, perceiving this arrangement as an attempt by nurses to capture their area of practice. However, careful explanation that this is designed to benefit the patient, for example, by performing certain exercises taught to him by the physiotherapist three times a day for seven days a week instead of five days, makes the intentions and benefits of the system apparent to the patient.

As none of the paramedical staff is part of the unit's nursing structure, they continue to wear white coats or uniforms. Some therapists feel unable to treat a patient unless they have had a referral from a doctor. This is potentially a problem as the doctor might not visit for several days. In the unit the problem was overcome by the medical staff providing a 'blanket' referral covering all patients to the units, so those requiring specialist therapy can receive it at the earliest opportunity.

THE MULTIDISCIPLINARY CLINICAL TEAM (MDCT)

The multidisciplinary clinical team comprises of the patient and his family, and all workers contributing to his health care (McFarlane, 1980). The concept of teamwork, rather than working as a group of individuals is seen as an important factor in the care of patients in the nursing development units: 'The primary objective of any team function, therefore, is to coordinate the health care given by different contributors to an individual which might otherwise remain uncoordinated or even in conflict.' Before members work as a team it is advantageous for each member to understand the roles of the other team members, and how they perceive that role. To facilitate that process the multidisciplinary clinical team is asked to participate in experiential learning. This involves representatives of several disciplines. By using a video camera to record interactions between various team members and actors playing the roles of patients the remaining team members are able to observe both the unique and the routine fields of practice of the disciplines involved. This method, described by Pearson, Morris and Whitehouse (1985) has an added advantage in that the actor can stay in role and later provide perceptions of what has occurred from the recipient of the care.

The keyworker

A team benefits from a leader, and in the case of the multidisciplinary clinical team in hospital, this position has traditionally been held by a medical consultant. However, in the NDUs where the primary need of the patients is for nursing the nurse practitioner coordinates the plans and decisions of the team.

The rationale for this leadership of the team by the patient's 'keyworker' in the discipline involved can be easily demonstrated. In 1966 Henderson showed how the contributions made to patient care by various disciplines can be represented by the segments of a circle, the whole circle representing the total professional health care input to the patient. In some settings it is possible that a discipline may have little or no role, such as the occupational therapist in an intensive therapy unit. However, in most settings one discipline can be identified as making the largest contribution. For example, in the NDUs where patients are admitted with a major requirement for nursing, and where primary nursing provides a professional nurse who has a close therapeutic relationship with the patient, it seems reasonable to identify the nurse practitioner as the 'keyworker'.

McFarlane (1980) suggests that the keyworker should lead the team, stating that: 'If the major objective of a clinical team is to coordinate the plans of care evolved by different health workers, then it would seem logical that the member of the team taking major responsibility for the care of the individual should be in the leadership position.' Clearly as team-leader the nurse does not direct the other health care workers, rather she coordinates and harmonises care by helping create common goals between the health professionals and the patient.

The review

The multidisciplinary review is held once a week on the unit, with all members of the team present. Each nurse practitioner presents the patients (who may choose to be present) and leads the discussion. It is the responsibility of the nurse practitioner to summarise the consensus feeling of the team and to ensure that all decisions are recorded.

THE MANAGEMENT OF PATIENT INFORMATION

The communication of patient information is a complicated

Figure 3.2 The Communications Maze. Patient-related information from both outside and inside the hospital must pass through the maze to the patient. Workers at openings need not necessarily convey the information beyond that point themselves, but must be aware of what information has passed through.

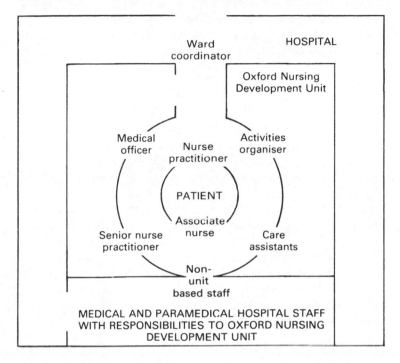

process in a hospital, often involving many different workers. The routes for such communication for incoming patient-centred information is represented by the 'communication maze' (Figure 3.2). This shows how information about the patient from either outside or inside the hospital enters the units in only two ways. The first is via the ward coordinator, who either passes the information direct to the nurse on duty, or via the medical officer or senior nurse practitioner. Unqualified staff, such as care assistants or the activities organiser, are not valid routes for patient communication. Alternatively, information may go direct to non-unit-based staff such as the social worker who has direct access to the units. Obviously if the social worker, for example, wishes to convey that information direct to the patient she can do so, as long as the nurse as keyworker is made aware of what has been said, perhaps at the multidisciplinary review.

Written information about the patient is either kept in the patient's medical notes, or more often in the nursing notes. Other disciplines such as social work and occupational therapy contribute directly to these notes, which are open to the patient and (with his permission) his family.

STAFFING PATTERNS

The ratio of eight patients to each nurse practitioner has already been mentioned. The units both have two primary nurses, each having a team of associate nurses who provide care in her absence. At any time only one nurse from each team is on duty to provide direct care to the patients. Occasionally an overlap brings the number of nurses on duty up to three, which releases one of the primary nurses to fulfil her teaching or research responsibilities, or to go on a home assessment with a patient.

Nurse practitioners (that is, primary nurses) generally work from 8.00 to 4.30 five days a week, including alternate weekends. Each nurse practitioner has a full-time associate who covers her days off and evenings. All other evenings and night duty are filled by part-time associates. As the associate nurses always care for the same nurse practitioner's patients, it is possible for a patient to be nursed by only six different people during his whole admission. When this is compared with the number of nurses who care for a patient day and night on a ward run on the traditional system the opportunity for developing close nurse–patient relationships under primary nursing is clear. Furthermore, both associate nurses and nurse practitioners have an opportunity to understand each other's professional practices and attitudes.

Apart from the two nurses on duty each shift, a number of care assistants are available during the day. In the morning two work from 7.30 to 2.00, and one from 9.00 to 4.00. In the evening two care assistants are on duty between 5.00 and 10.00. Care assistants are not formally attached to a nurse practitioner; however, they are allocated on a daily basis. Therefore, in the morning a care assistant will be allocated to each nurse who will briefly inform her of the assistance she will require during her span of duty (such as, for example, bathing a patient at 10.00). This not only allows the care assistant to plan her other work in advance around the needs of the patients, but also to anticipate the work of the nurse, in this case by running the bath and taking the patient's towels and toiletries to the bathroom at 9.55.

Finally there is a ward coordinator on duty between 9.00 and 4.00, and 4.00 and 8.00 pm seven days a week, providing a constant filter for the nurses. At night, two associates are on duty.

These staffing levels, utilising all registered nurses and care assistants, is extremely cost effective, saving £30 000 per annum (1985–86 estimates) when compared with a similar ward. This finding is in line with studies from other countries (Fagin, 1982; LaForme, 1982).

FORMAL UNIT-BASED STAFF COMMUNICATION

Staff council

The atmosphere in the units is non-hierarchical and encourages free speech between members. Therefore, decisions about the running of the unit are made at monthly staff council meetings. Any member of staff may attend these, including care assistants and ward coordinators, and while there is a prearranged agenda any subject may be brought up for discussion, and if a decision is required it may be put to a vote of the council. Minutes of the meetings are subsequently circulated to all staff.

Staff support group

Punton (1985) describes stress experienced by primary nurses at Burford Community Hospital. Any member of staff may be subject to stress; for example, associate nurses having to work unsupervised and independently may express feelings of isolation. Therefore, a staff support group was set up and a counsellor from outside the hospital invited to lead the sessions. This method has been used successfully for many years in high technology units such as intensive therapy units or renal units

(Jackson, 1980). Webster *et al*. (1982) have described many positive outcomes from such a group, such as increased social interaction, peer support at work, and participation in ward meetings.

Staff seminars

Motivation amongst all nursing staff to extend their knowledge has been consistently high on the unit. Therefore monthly staff seminars are held to share knowledge between nurses. These may take various forms: perhaps one month care planning is discussed and original care plans examined; another month nurses who have been to conferences feed back their impressions of the conference to the rest of the staff and describe the major points discussed. All nurses are invited to choose a nursing topic in which they are interested, and to act as a resource person to the rest of the staff, with some nurses leading seminars on their chosen topic.

CONCLUSION

In this chapter the implementation of primary nursing in the Burford and Oxford nursing development units has been described, showing that the reported gap between theory and practice can be bridged. One of the key aspects is that not only has the nursing structure been changed, but also that ancillary support to the nurses on the ward has been modified. By introducing a system that allows qualified professional nurses to practise nursing it is possible for nurses to be accountable for the care of a group of patients. This is not substituting nurses for the doctors who have traditionally led care teams, rather it is implementing consensus decision-making by the whole team with the nurse coordinating those decisions. The concept of authoritarian leadership has been abandoned, not only in the management of patient care, but also in the treatment of staff, who are encouraged to influence decisions about the ward through such means as the staff council.

The Burford and Oxford nursing development units have been a major development in the implementation of primary nursing in this country, however as isolated units they may be regarded as an oddity. It is only if they have the effect of a catalyst in that primary nursing becomes more widely introduced that their true value will be realised.

REFERENCES

Bergman, R. (1981) 'Accountability — Definition and Dimensions'. *International Nursing Review*, 28(2), 53–59.

DeCarlo, T.J. (1974) 'Recreation Participation Patterns and Successful Ageing'. *Journal of Gerontology*, 29(4), 416–422.

Fagin, C.M. (1982) 'The Economic Value'. *American Journal of Nursing*, December, 1844–1849.

Ford, L.C. (1979) 'A Nurse for All Settings: The Nurse Practitioner'. *Nursing Outlook*, 27(8), 516–521.

Henderson, V. (1966) *The Nature of Nursing*. (Collier Macmillan, London).

Jackson, V. (1980) 'Reducing Job Stress by Open Meetings'. *Nephrology Nurse*, November–December, 32–34.

LaForme, S. (1982) 'Primary Nursing: Does It Cost More?' *The Canadian Nurse*, April, 42–49.

McFarlane, J. (1980) 'The Multi-disciplinary Team', in Batchelor, I. and McFarlane, J. (eds) *Multidisciplinary Clinical Teams*. (Kings Fund Centre, London).

Manthey, M. (1970) 'The History and Development of Primary Nursing'. *Nursing Forum*, 9(4), 358–379.

Manthey, M. (1973) 'Primary Nursing is Alive and Well in the Hospital'. *American Journal of Nursing*, 73(1), 83–87.

Manthey, M. (1980) *The Practice of Primary Nursing*. (Blackwells, Oxford).

Miller, A. (1985) 'The Relationship Between Nursing Theory and Nursing Practice'. *Journal of Advanced Nursing*, 10(5), 417–429.

Pearson, A. (1984) 'The Burford Experience'. *Nursing Mirror*, 159(22), 32–35.

Pearson, A., Morris, P. and Whitehouse, C. (1985) 'Consumer-oriented Groups: A New Approach to Interdisciplinary Teaching'. *Journal of the Royal College of General Practitioners*, August, 381–383.

Pembrey, S. (1984) 'Nursing Care: Professional Progress'. *Journal of Advanced Nursing*, 9, 539–547.

Punton, S. (1985) 'Coping with Primary nursing'. *Nursing Times*, 2 January, 50.

Roper, N., Tierney, N. and Logan, W. (1985) *The Elements of Nursing*, 2nd edn. (Churchill Livingstone, Edinburgh).

Silver, H.K., Ford, L.C., Ripley, S.S. and Isoe, J. (1985) 'Perspectives Twenty Years Later. From the Pioneers of the Nurse Practitioner Movement'. *Nurse Practitioner*, 10(1), 15–18.

Webster, S., Kelly, L.A., Johst, B., Weber, R. and Wickes, L. (1982) 'The Support Group'. *Nursing Management*, 13(9), 26–30.

4

Nursing Beds and Nursing Therapy

Steven Ersser

INTRODUCTION

The nursing development units provide beds for patients whose primary need is for nursing. They are essentially nursing-oriented and the focus of care is therapeutic nursing, as outlined in the other chapters of this book. The notion of nursing beds is quite new in Britain, and only one centre is known in the United States. To explore this topic fully, it is necessary to analyse the nature of hospital care and therapeutic nursing in some depth.

If you were admitted to a hospital tomorrow invariably your admission for 'medical care' would have to be sanctioned by a doctor; as such, you will end up in a 'medical bed'. Throughout your stay your assigned diagnosis will be the predominant factor guiding where you go and what happens to you. This is despite the fact that your health needs are likely to be multiple and complex — going far beyond the picture of pathology identified (if any exists at all!).

There are important weaknesses in this assumption. Many people requiring inpatient care either do not have a significant need for a medical service, or if they do this is often required principally during the short, acute phase of illness. However, in the immediate recovery phase up to discharge these patients remain in the acute-medical setting, where there are many obstacles to the patient's full range of health needs being met because the priority has to be given to those who are in acute need. This may present difficulties for those in the recovery-rehabilitative phase of their illness who are adjusting perhaps to the stress of treatment, the acute environment and the emotional and social consequences of these changes. By necessity the medical and nursing staff are preoccupied with helping those patients whose condition is physiologically unstable and potentially life-threatening. Here the nurse's collaborative role with the doctor is particularly active — carrying out the treatment plans and monitoring its effect on the patient.

It is argued here that those people who have a predominant need for intensive nursing, and whose condition is sufficiently stable such that they do not require frequent contact with medical staff, would be likely to benefit most in a nursing unit where nursing becomes the fundamental therapy, supported by the multidisciplinary team.

ARE HEALTH NEEDS ALWAYS MEDICAL NEEDS?

The underlying issue is whether or not health and medical needs are always one or the same thing. Despite traditional emphasis in practice this is not always the case.

Those patients entering the immediate recovery phase of their illness, and some patients directly admitted to the ward who are 'medically' stable, do not always necessarily have an intensive definitive need for the medical service. Such patients are often likely to have some of the following health needs.

- Help to adjust to the stress of their illness (whether defined or not), their treatment or the limitations of age or handicap, and their emotional and social consequences.
- The need to acquire the knowledge, skills and confidence to regain and retain their maximum level of independence through guidance and teaching.
- The need to receive comfort and support that enhance the adjustments described.
- Help for those who are dependent in those 'self-care' activities such as washing, moving and eating.
- The essential need for 'care' not 'cure' in those people who are terminally ill.
- Help for those people with ill-defined conditions who continue to feel ill (a common problem since illness as opposed to disease is socially defined; Field, 1976).

61

WHY PEOPLE ARE IN NEED OF HOSPITAL CARE

The reason for hospital admission will usually follow the prevailing morbidity and demographic pattern. The increasing trend in the prevalence of chronic illness and disability is a consequence of factors such as greater longevity and a growing elderly population (DHSS, 1976, 1978b, 1981; Doyal, 1979). The *Hospital In-patient Enquiry* (DHSS, 1985b) provides some indication of cause for hospital admission — reflected as 10 per cent of conditions on death and discharge. The largest group was those patients with ill-defined conditions, followed by cardiovascular disease, injury, poisoning, diseases of the digestive and respiratory systems, and malignant neoplasms — many of these conditions are chronic in nature. Medical diagnosis is only a guide to the health needs of the inpatient population, particularly those with a chronic illness; here nurses are particularly well placed to help (Diers, 1981; Hockey, 1978).

THE LIMITATIONS OF THE HOSPITAL MEDICAL SERVICE IN MEETING HEALTH NEEDS

The foregoing description of health needs for the hospitalised patient reflects the limitations of current medical practice. Contrary to popular belief this has been the case throughout history where 'medicine' has in many areas failed to meet society's health needs as a whole as evidenced by the work of Dubos (1959), McKeown (1976), Illich (1976), and Doyal (1979), who describe how most ill-health is caused by a complex effect of environment and human behaviour which often limits the use of simple 'cures'. Further, there are indications that much illness and patient dependency is aggravated by the medical service (Illich, 1976; Miller, 1985a).

Campbell (1984) has said: 'We can view medical power as the successful dominance of the health care service by one profession whose claims to effectiveness is in truth poorly founded.' Capra (1982) supports this argument. It has been said that the genuine power of medicine stems from its capacity to identify and cooperate with healing forces already present in the person, social group or environment (Friedson, 1975; Kennedy, 1981; Campbell, 1984).

The powerful influence of the biomedical model has served as a conceptual straitjacket for health workers by confining their thinking in terms of disease rather than health. The deep-seated cartesian-reductionist view of man identifies him as analogous to a machine, a composite of parts. The contrasting paradigm is the holistic model which considers man to be greater than the sum of his parts. As such, illness is viewed as a disorder of a particular tissue or organ rather than an adverse change in the person's total situation.

Medicine has been protected by a cloak of mystique arising from the process of high level specialisation and categorisation of disease (Capra, 1982). Furthermore the sharing of knowledge has been restricted, particularly between doctors and laymen (Berger and Luckmann, 1971; Kalisch, 1979).

The medical service can magnify the obstruction it imposes to meeting health needs by limiting the effectiveness of other health workers. This is perhaps primarily achieved by the all-pervasive influence of the biomedical model and attempting to maintain a monopoly of knowledge about disease and health. Capra (1982) has said that this has unfairly thrown into question the efficacy of other health workers. This has been seen recently in the BMA report on alternative medicine (Veitch, 1986). This has been the case for several centuries, says Versluysen (1980) who identifies the neglect throughout English history of the impact of women healers. Strategies exist in practice which continue to deny nurses expression of their expertise on health matters (Thomstad, 1975; Stein 1978).

Nurses are increasingly realising the inadequacy of the medical diagnosis as the primary directive of nursing need (Tierney, 1984) and the tradition of the recent past on the focus of nursing on disease and task rather than the patient (Baly, 1975, 1980). The effectiveness of the nursing service has been confined by the continuous delegation of unwanted medical tasks; this in turn has led to the relegation of nursing itself to the hands of the untrained in practice (Rogers, 1972; Bellaby and Oribabor, 1980). However, it is often forgotten that 'the nurse's primary responsibility is to those people who require nursing care' (ICN, 1973).

HEALTH NEEDS OF THE HOSPITAL PATIENT: WHAT THE NURSING SERVICE HAS TO OFFER

The question arises as to what nurses have to offer those people admitted to hospital which is not provided by the medical service.

The list of health needs described on p.61 are those which the nursing service commonly attempts to meet. The domain of nursing practice is reflected in various nursing models. A recurrent theme in models popular in Britain is that which emphasises the nurse's concern with everyday self-care activity, normally carried out unaided by the patient (Henderson, 1960; Orem, 1980; Roper, Logan and Tierney, 1980). Despite the value of considering an explicit model of practice, Orem (1980) has said that it is a feature of effective nurses to recognise when people are in need of nursing.

Nursing need has also been conceptualised as the need for care. Leininger (1984) has described care broadly in terms of arts which ameliorate or improve the human condition. Many have argued that nurses have relegated their caring role and so it is in this area that the role needs expansion (Pembrey, 1979; McFarlane, 1980; Leininger, 1985; Kitson, 1985). The importance of this role when the curative approach is no longer appropriate has been stressed in government reports (Briggs, 1972; Merrison, 1979).

Wilson-Barnett (1984) has made a more pragmatic attempt to isolate the key nursing functions:

● understanding illness and treatment from the patient's viewpoint;
● providing continuous psychological care during illness and critical events;
● helping people cope with illness or potential health problems;
● providing comfort; and
● coordinating treatments and other events affecting the patient.

In many ways it seems ironic that nurses, the largest collective of health workers in this country, have not up to now been able to present to society the extensive service they can offer, particularly for those having a primary requirement for them. Perhaps we are moving in this direction with greater educational developments and the subsequent clarification and analysis of the service that nurses provide. Orem (1980) has argued for the need of society to provide ways and means to bring people in need of nursing in contact with qualified nurses.

At present people are usually deemed to require hospital care through medical assessment on point of entry. Contact is made with the nursing service through entry to ward or clinic typically organised on the basis of medical need. Of course, by necessity, there are many areas where nursing and medical services must collaborate closely, but not all.

INDEPENDENT NURSING PRACTICE FOR THOSE WHOSE MAIN NEED IS FOR NURSING

Certain areas exist within current NHS provision for those people predominantly needing the nursing service. The nursing home provides a permanent home placement where nursing and supervision are required to maintain a state of rehabilitation which the patient's potential allows (Wade, Sawyer and Bell, 1983). This provision developed because of the large number of elderly people requiring long-stay hospital beds (DHSS, 1978b). The medical needs of nursing home residents are met by general practitioners. Wade, Sawyer and Bell's (1983) extensive study was intended as a basis for policy review. It identified many anomalies in the present system of care for the elderly requiring ongoing care — such as dependency level being poorly matched with their location. Alternative models of care were explored — with the Danish system of nurse-led units proving to be the most promising. The DHSS (1985a) paper, *Experimental NHS Houses for Elderly People*, describes three trial schemes where the care provided will continue to be principally nursing in nurse-led homes in the public sector.

Before describing other areas of independent practice it is necessary to distinguish between the extension and expansion of the nurse's role, which is often confused in the literature. Role extension refers to a situation where nursing expertise is not vital, and where the additional tasks incorporated into the widened role are essentially medical (MacGuire, 1980); such changes have largely taken place in North America to compensate for shortages of physicians (Morgan, 1972), and some have considered this as a misuse of nursing resource (Schlotfeldt, 1972). In contrast, role expansion emphasises the 'deepening' and development of the skills and knowledge which is uniquely nursing (Pearson, 1983); often both roles are combined. These combined roles have been seen in the nurse practitioner movement in North America although the original intention (which still remains in some areas) is for a role presenting the essential nature of nursing. Much confusion and anxiety by the medical profession about autonomous nursing practice has arisen because of failure to differentiate role extension and expansion; this confusion has been typified by Mitchell (1984).

Few known areas exist of independent nursing practice which adopt an expanded role. This includes the independent nursing clinic (Kinlein and Young, 1977), in contrast to clinics where nurses have an extended role such as the arthritis clinic described by Hill (1985).

The provision of nursing beds for patients and their families requiring 24 hour professional nursing exist in three known centres: the Loeb Center for Nursing and Rehabilitation, Montefiore Hospital, New York; Burford Community Hospital, Oxford; and Beeson Ward (Oxford nursing development unit), Radcliffe Infirmary, Oxford.

THE REQUIREMENTS FOR AUTONOMOUS PRACTICE

Nurses must be allowed to practise more autonomously if they are to provide society with the service of nursing beds. Autonomy, the authority to determine or regulate one's own acts without outside interference, is granted when society is confident that an occupation has specialised knowledge and skills for the service of the community (Jacox, 1978). The presence of such skills gives nurses this authority (RCN, 1976).

Whether in autonomous practice or not the nurse is accountable to her patients. This in turn requires that she receives the corresponding authority and responsibility (RCN, 1981). In a nursing unit the nurse practitioner not the medical consultant is legally responsible for the overall care of the patient. Their normal level of accountability remains, but the sensitive awareness of the need to make the referrals to other experts, particularly medical staff, is essential. Each individual nurse, as always, remains accountable for the care she gives (Rowden, 1984). This legal requirement sufficiently covers the operations of nurses in the British nursing units.

Another necessity is the need for the direct access of nurses to patients and vice versa. Norris (1970) criticises the single control of entry into and pathway through the hospital by doctors. This does not necessarily mean that nurses have primary therapeutic responsibility, but it certainly does not negate it.

Some of the means by which nurse–patient access has been restricted lie in the organisation of hospital care and the biomedical ethos. The legal position also appears to have its restrictions. Telford (1985) describes how a nurse is usually employed under a 'contract of services' making her accountable to her superiors. This differs from medical consultants who are employed under a 'contract for services' which allows freedom in clinical judgement. The imposition here for nurses, however, may really be that of the bureaucratic organisation, based on hierarchical lines. Primary nursing provides the framework for exercising clear lines of accountability and freedom in clinical judgement.

THE EFFECTIVENESS OF NURSING BEDS

Studies in evaluation

Studies of both patient outcome, quality of care and economic situation of each of the three existing locations with nursing beds are summarised in Table 4.1.

Collectively, the evidence suggests that for patients meeting the admission (study) criteria the patient outcome experience is positive, the quality assurance scores are high and the running costs are low — relative to that of a comparable patient group cared for in an acute unit of a conventional hospital. Results of the Oxford nursing development unit study are unavailable as yet. The findings of this study should have great significance for the hospital nursing service. The stringency of the research design is greater with a larger sample and setting the nursing unit within a conventional district-type hospital.

The effectiveness of nurses working in autonomous practice

Various studies indicate that nurses in general function effectively in terms of patient outcome and cost in other types of

Table 4.1 Indicators of the Effectiveness of Nursing Beds

Location of nursing beds	Effect on patients			Quality assurance tests		Economic considerations
	Patient outcome studies					
	Methodology	Results and significance	Study reference	Nursing audit* (Phaneuf, 1976)	Quality of patient care scale Qualpacs** (Wandelt and Ager, 1974)	
1. Loeb Centre	*Aim*: to compare the patient outcome of the hospitalisation of a group of patients at Loeb with a comparable group (control) nursed in a conventional hospital. *Sample*: Those meeting Loeb's admission criteria: (1) evidence of favourable prognosis for return to community; (2) previous Loeb admission; (3) medical diagnosis of community importance. *Design: Experimental* The sample were randomised into study control group and comparability control measures	Loeb patients were (1) less frequently hospitalised; (2) if they were it was after a longer period than the control group; (3) more likely to return to work and social activities; (4) comparable with control group in functional ability and mortality states. The report could not conclude that the differing experiences were due to	Hall *et al.* (1975)	Not assessed	Not assessed	Hall *et al.* (1975) found that the average stay at Loeb was 5.5 days greater than the control hospital, *but* this was at lower cost. The report highlights that the long-term benefits of significantly lower readmission rates following a longer period after discharge at Loeb are considerable.

were applied to ensure that differences in outcome were attributable to different nursing environments.	the nursing experience alone.			
2. Burford Hospital	*Aim*: broadly — to describe the effects of introducing a 'new ideology' of nursing (reflecting the 'expanded' professional role in the Burford nursing unit). Changes: (1) systematic care planning; (2) primary nursing; (3) partnership with patients; (4) open records; (5) flexible patient day; (6) qualified nurses giving care; (7) community involvement in unit. *Design*: (A) *Action research*: used to describe and analyse the process of change when the new practices were established. (B) *Experimental phase*: to test the generated hypothesis that the practice norms in the nursing unit differed from those in other hospitals and that these would directly improve patient outcomes. *Sample*: 64 patients admitted to three nursing beds with either a fractured neck of femur or abdominal hysterectomy.	Burford (experimental) patients were: (1) more satisfied with their life in general (life satisfaction index); (2) more satisfied with their care than the control group (satisfaction with care index). In the nursing dependency index: Burford patients had lower dependency scores on average; all three items were not significant on chi-square test — however it is clear that patients admitted to nursing beds experienced positive outcome effects. Pearson (1985a & b)	Of the 16 Burford patient records assessed all were in the 'good' or 'excellent' quality of care categories; of the 47 control patient records assessed 34 per cent entered into those two categories	For the Burford nursing unit Qualpac scores rose from 'below average' to 'almost excellent' as a result of the changes taking place. No assessment performed in control hospital.	Pearson (1985a) found that the running costs of a nursing unit compared to a conventional one were cheaper for three main reasons: (1) lower starting costs because of high ancillary/ support staff-to-nurse ratio; (2) medical cover by general practitioner; (3) long-term savings from lower readmission rates.

* Use of nursing records   ** Use of observation

Table 4.1 (continued)

Location of nursing beds	Effect on patients					Economic considerations
	Patient outcome studies		Study reference	Quality assurance tests		
	Methodology	Results and significance		Nursing audit* (Phaneuf, 1976)	Quality of patient care scale Qualpacs** (Wandelt and Ager, 1974)	
3. Oxford Nursing Development Unit (Beeson ward)	An ongoing study taking place in 16 nursing beds on Beeson Aim: as that of the Loeb study (above) (study/experimental patients on Beeson) — to study the effect of intensive nursing on patient outcomes. Sample: (1) over 60 years; (2) admitted to an acute hospital with either (a) fractured neck of femur, (b) cerebrovascular accident, (c) lower limb amputation, (d) abdominal hysterectomy; (3) independent enough in activities of living to enable them to live in their own home or part III home; (4) is rational and orientated (to be able to participate in the study); (5) discharge back to the community	Data unavailable as yet	Pearson (1985b	Of the 26 audits performed so far, all were in the excellent category (Bradshaw, 1986).	Although no formal assessments have been performed either at ONDU or control units there are two indicative studies carried out on Beeson. (1) First by two teams of two nurse observers on a quality	Unavailable as yet but two factors remain which will have a tendency to make running costs cheaper. (1) Part-time medical staff (one houseman) on Beeson for 16 patients. (2) High ancillary/support staff-to-nurse ratio.

should be a feasible possibility; (6) medical assessment reveals that no major medical conditions exist requiring acute hospital care; (7) nursing assessment should indicate a need for nursing on the CAPE (Clifton Assessment Procedures for the Elderly scale; see Pattie (1981) and Pattie and Gilleard (1975).

Design: as Loeb study. Tools (1) the dependency index, (2) life and care satisfaction indices. Medical staff are asked to make a referral to the unit for patients eligible for inclusion. Once medical and nursing assessments have taken place, randomisation occurs. Control patients follow the normal pattern of hospitalisation — either remaining in the acute unit or transferred to a community hospital.
Data collection: at discharge + at six weeks + six months post discharge. References for tools used in discharge schedule:

(1) the patient service checklist (Hall et al., 1975).
(2) the life satisfaction profile (Neugarten, Harighurst and Tobin, 1961; Luker, 1982).
(3) the dependency index (Garraway et al., 1980).

assurance training course. Result: best care category; (2) By a MSc research student assessing one nurse only on a 'busy morning'. Results: 'just below best category' (Bradshaw, 1986).

* Use of nursing records   ** Use of observation

independent practice. In contrast to the nursing bed studies those described here involve nurses working in an extended role context, or with a mixture of role extension and expansion.

Nurse practitioners working within an inpatient rehabilitation setting compared favourably with physician-managed patients with six medical conditions (Weinberg, Liljestraud and Moore, 1983). Nurses achieved a slightly shorter length of stay and a higher 'condition index score' with lower investigation costs, although the nurses had half the caseload of the physician. Although no statistical difference exists the researchers claim that the findings are consistent with the effectiveness of nurses in outpatient settings. Macauley and Anderson's (1974) study of the nurse as a primary therapist with stroke patients describes a comparable degree of effectiveness compared with team care — but at a significantly lower cost. Nurses have had a significant success in caring independently for nursing home residents and in the community (Sackett et al., 1977).

NURSING AS A THERAPY

> Nurses must be able to define what activities they perform and how these affect society.
>
> Gingell (1985)

A broad look will now be taken at the general approaches nurses use to help those with health needs, followed by a description of therapeutic nursing approaches which have the potential to enhance a patient's wellbeing.

Nursing approaches to helping people

Dorethea Orem (1980) has described the different types of skilled help that nurses can offer society: acting or doing for; teaching; guiding and supporting (comforting); and providing an environment that promotes personal development in relation to meeting present or future demands for action. Skill is also needed in uniquely selecting and applying these methods to each individual. Although they are often used when the nurse is helping the person with self-care activities, the former often uses them interchangeably. For example, while helping wash a stroke patient, the nurse will partly be 'doing for', teaching and guiding, and may also provide physical comfort giving the opportunity to help the patient express his/her anxieties and thereby perhaps offload some of his/her emotional discomfort. Through providing help in all these ways, the nurse can help a patient adjust and cope with his/her past, present and future situation, the final aim being to make the person independent of nursing help altogether. Another fundamental objective of nursing is to help people feel better as well as get better. Whether purposeful or not, the approaches used by nurses which produce such benefits constitute the use of nursing as a therapy.

Historical recognition

'Therapy' has been described as that which 'attends' to the healing process (Capra, 1982). Observation that some positive change or 'healing effect' in the patient often takes place, whether measurable or subjectively experienced by patient or nurse, when the patient receives nursing care leads to the premise that nursing itself may be exerting a therapeutic effect.

Historically nurses have 'applied' the medical therapy of patients. However, it has often been assumed that improvement in his condition is solely due to his drugs or surgery. This causal relationship is questionable when the patient's care has also involved the potent variable — the 24 hour contact of nurse and patient, offering comfort, rest, good food and drink and a listening ear — to name but a few subtle influences. It is these methods and effects that nurses must explore.

There are early indications of the recognition of 'nursing and therapy'. Nightingale (1859/1980) pointed out that while then (as now) the efficacy of many medical therapies had not been ascertained: 'there is universal experience as to the extreme importance of careful nursing in determining the issue of disease'. To date the English history of healing has concerned itself with organised medicine, while the integral role of woman healers in caring for society's sick has been neglected. Before the late seventeenth century, the impact of medicine on everyday healing experience was minimal. As few doctors existed prior to the eighteenth century health needs were mainly met by women through their sheer numbers and practical experience of healing (Versluysen, 1980). Capra (1982) adds that 'the important role that nurses play in the healing process through their human contact with patients is not fully realised'.

Recognition of a nurse's therapeutic effect has been described by Travelbee (1966) who talked of the 'therapeutic use of self'. She believed that the conscious use of the nurse's personality and knowledge could 'effect a change in the ill person (which) alleviates the individual's distress'.

It would seem to be a feature of nursing activity that it has a potentially positive effect on people. Many medical therapies, although often of benefit, also incidentally inflict discomfort and other unwanted effects. Therapeutic nursing could perhaps describe those approaches used by nurses which have an over-riding tendency to produce subjective feelings of improvement in the person being helped, whether or not a demonstrable change is evident.

A philosophy of nursing

The effect nurses have on patients will be influenced by their philosophy of nursing which in turn will shape the form in which the nurse–patient contact is expressed. Such a philosophy is a reflection of what the nurse believes and values about nursing. Prophit (1986) has emphasised the necessity of such a philosophy for clinical nurses as a practical prerequisite for an effective nursing service. A philosophy based on a concept of care, valuing commitment, skills and knowledge, and respect for persons are components of nursing whose synthesis has been described as constituting therapeutic nursing activity (Kitson, 1985). A philosophy of care for nurses as a means to 'improve the human condition' has also been expressed by Leininger (1985).

Therapeutic approaches in nursing

Five broad categories of therapeutic approaches in nursing are described:

● The nurse–patient relationship
● Creating a therapeutic environment

● Giving information
● Providing comfort
● Holistic health practices.

The nurse–patient relationship

The potential of the nurse to help another lies in the relationship between them which is at the heart of the helping situation. It not only provides the milieu for expressing therapeutic methods, but has itself the potential to serve therapeutic effect (Peplau, 1952; Travelbee, 1966; Hall, 1969; Jourard, 1971; Hall *et al.*, 1975). Cormack (1985) describes the psychotherapeutic use of the relationship in which 'the nurse uses her warmth, personality, understanding of human behaviour, empathy and communication skills in order to help the individual'.

The complexities of the relationship are not described here; however, a description of Lydia Hall's theory of how it may be effective is given as an example. Hall's work has had a significant influence on the philosophy of nursing in the development units.

The influence of Lydia Hall and Carl Rogers. Lydia Hall was director of the Loeb Center for Nursing, the world's first known unit of its type. Stevens (1979) said that Hall was in fact a powerful theorist although she would probably not identify herself as such, and that Hall's theory was a good example of an extant theory — one that has high potential for application to practice. Her concept of nursing focused on nursing as a therapy.

Hall (1969) believed that nurses could aid healing by helping people to learn. She valued a patient's autonomy as reflected in practice by a philosophy of partnership with the patients at Loeb: 'Patients were the achievers and . . . nurses . . . the facilitators, teachers, supporters and nurturers' (Hall *et al.*, 1975; Figure 4.1).

She felt that the prerequisites to support this learning were uniquely offered by the nurse through combined concern with the person ('the core'), his disease ('the cure'), and the provision of nurture ('the care') (see Figure 4.1). Hall thought the adjustment when recovering from illness (particularly chronic illness) or disability often involved an adjustment of lifestyle which depended on an affective change.

75

Figure 4.1 A Diagrammatic Representation of Lydia Hall's Beliefs about the Therapeutic Effect of Nursing, based on Hall (1959). The 'core' = the person; the 'care' = the body (representing nurture — intimate bodily care); the 'cure' = the disease: seeing the patient and family through the medical aspects of nursing.

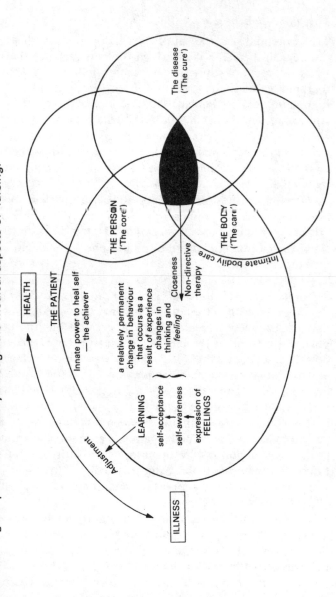

Hall said that nurses could help people adjust in this way using the provision of intimate physical care in which the nurse is often engaged. She believed (1969, p. 10) that 'the exclusive aspect of nursing is the nurturing one'.

This fundamental 'nurture' or 'care' aspect of nursing was seen to serve three purposes:

● helping the person through guiding and 'doing for';
● providing comfort; and
● fostering the helping relationship (the 'core' of nursing) through facilitating closeness with the patient.

Hall felt that when this took place the patient's exploration and expression of his feelings was more likely. When people are carrying out everyday activities with the nurse their limitations become obvious to them. But their self-awareness is deepened, aiding adjustment and therefore health because, Hall argued, changes in behaviour rely fundamentally on a change of feelings rather than of thought (Hall, 1964, 1969).

The thinking of Lydia Hall has clearly been influenced by that of the psychotherapist Carl Rogers. Rogers (1951) describes his theory of personality and behaviour. The Rogerian influence is currently highlighted by the writing of Genrose Alfano (1985), current director of Loeb. One aspect of Rogerian thought was that an individual's behaviour is shaped by his goals which satisfy needs experienced in his perception of the world. These motives are accompanied by emotions. Rogers believed that people tend to move in a direction of maturation — but moving closer to their goals in a non-directive helping situation where the person is allowed to explore his own feelings and motives. The stress of Rogers on understanding a person's perception of his situation, and the limitations of trying to understand another from one's own external frame of reference, appears to be a concept increasingly valued by nurses.

The influence of the Loeb Center for Nursing is largely that of Lydia Hall herself. Her achievement in applying her own conception of nursing to practice, one envisaged to have direct therapeutic influence through the patient's contact with a nurse, is a substantial one in the development of nursing.

Creating a therapeutic environment

A feature of hospital care is that nurses are in constant contact with patients. Nurses not only share the same environment but are also largely responsible for shaping the physical and psychosocial setting in which healing takes place. Hall *et al.* (1975, p. 3) has described the nurse's concern to: 'manage the environment in which the patient is housed'. Although over 125 years ago Nightingale (1859/1980) observed:

. . . [nursing] has been limited to signify little more than the administration of medicines and the application of poultices. It ought to signify the proper use of fresh air, warmth, cleanliness, quiet and the proper selection and administration of diet all at least expense of the vital power to the patient . . . the symptoms or sufferings generally considered to be inevitable and incident to the disease are very often not symptoms of the disease at all.

In the units an attempt is made to create a homely environment in a normal ward in various ways. This includes the use of a carpeted sitting room, with soft lighting and hanging plants, and encouraging relatives to bring in some of the patient's personal belongings.

Some of the most powerful therapeutic effects nurses can exert on patients are through their effect on the organisation of the social environment. Nurses can do much to help alleviate the stress of the newly admitted patient whose anxiety is typically at its highest on admission (Franklin, 1974). Change in the environment itself can produce an adverse effect on the person (Roper, Logan and Tierney, 1980). At the units the aim is to offset this by allowing the patient to work out his/her 'pattern of day' with the nurse as a priority over often unnecessary routines. Other direct attempts to foster a healing setting are in the invitation for patients and staff to eat together, the nurses choosing not to wear uniforms, and the organisation of entertainments by the activities organiser.

Nursing which is organised to focus on the individual rather than on tasks and routines has been shown to be therapeutic (Kitson, 1984). This study complements Miller's (1985a) findings that the use of an individualised approach produced significantly lower patient dependency, allowed for a higher patient turnover, and improved the 'discharge-to-death ratio' compared with task-centred wards. Since primary nursing is by nature organised on patient-centred lines, it is predictable that its use will maximise the effects described. Further, Marram, Schlegel and Bens' (1974) study indicated that patients felt more satisfied with their nursing and felt more supported emotionally under a primary rather than a functional (task) nursing system.

The potential antitherapeutic effect of the hospital atmosphere can go unrecognised. Hospitals often feel, and perhaps are, both threatening and dehumanising environments (Mapa and Turner, 1979). Also, the general level of morale that pervades both hospital and wards can have an important bearing on patients and staff (Revans, 1964). Work continues at both Oxford and Burford nursing development units to create a relaxed, humane atmosphere in the ward setting, some of which has been captured by Levi (1985) and the *Daily Telegraph* (1986).

Giving information to patients and their families

That patients are often critical about poor information in hospital is well documented by the annual health ombudsman's reports and earlier studies (Cartwright, 1964; Raphael, 1969; Skeet, 1970). Titmuss (1958) said that: 'the barrier of silence is one element in a general failure to treat the patient'.

An inevitable consequence for the patient (and his family) is anxiety. Through the stress response he is not only likely to feel unpleasant, but may also suffer from the adverse physical effects on homeostasis and therefore recovery (Wilson-Barnett and Fordham, 1982).

Peplau (1960) believed that through purposefully talking with patients nurses could aid adjustment to their situation. Research evidence exists of the adjustment to critical events such as own investigation and surgery and the positive effect on patients' comfort and recovery by nurses carefully giving them information to aid adjustment (Hayward, 1975; Boore, 1978; Wilson-Barnett, 1978; Wilson-Barnett and Osborne, 1983; Davis, 1984). The outstanding problem now is that nurses are not using these findings (Davis, 1985).

Providing comfort

The need for comfort is universal. For the sick this is important not only to offset the discomfort of illness and anxieties, but also the adverse effects of the high technology hospital environment. Naisbitt (1984) has said that accompanying the development of technology in society there would be a counterbalancing trend towards growth of the human response. He identifies nursing itself, particularly primary nursing, as such a response.

The potential for providing comfort is bound up with most nursing activities, and its release often depends upon the relationship between nurse and patient and recognition of the need for comfort and opportunities to provide it.

Through giving information or altering the ward environment the nurse may produce comfort in the person, both mental and physical. Direct use of comfort measures includes: involving the patient in the assessment and management of his pain; the use of pillows and cushions; refreshing the patient; letting him enjoy a favourite piece of music, or comfort a visiting pet. Study of those comfort measures remains a rich pasture for research.

Holistic health practices

The distinction between the holistic view of the patient and the reductionist perspective has been described. From the literature it appears that a philosophy of nursing closely allied to that of holism is emerging. Capra (1982) has reinforced this. Holistic health practices emphasise the relationship between helper and the helped, and ecological considerations and the provision of measures to make people 'heal' and 'feel' better. In many respects, therefore, this embraces almost all therapeutic nursing approaches.

Krieger (1981) has offered a more specific description: 'The common denominator is that the practice allows the individual to explore and thereby become more aware of self. This is done by an inward focussing and persistent search for subtle cues to latent facets of consciousness that can be brought more fully into awareness.' They include:

● those practices rebalancing energy (such as acupuncture and acupressure);
● naturopathic medicine (such as therapeutic touch);
● therapy directed to the relationship between body and environment (such as therapeutic massage and stress reduction methods); and
● measures promoting self-awareness (such as art therapy).

The use of therapeutic touch has been chosen for discussion. Its practice has been of interest to nurses in the units. Therapeutic touch is a practice closely related to the method of nursing whereby people are nurtured using the hands to promote wellbeing.

Therapeutic touch. The motive of the nurse to touch a patient is often instrumental in physical care, although an expressive use which is effective and often spontaneous in nature may be used to convey compassion, understanding and empathy. LeMay's (1986) ongoing study of nurse–patient touch indicates that of 130 long-stay patients approximately 85 per cent was of an instrumental nature. Therapeutic touch is characterised by 'the touching of another in an act that incorporates an intent to help or heal the person so touched' (Krieger, 1981).

Krieger believes that physical contact through the normal energy field surrounding the person constitutes touch. Her studies began in 1972, with two replication studies in 1973 and 1974. She reported a significant change in haemoglobin and haematocrit levels from pretreatment values in the experimental group to a high confidence level ($p < 0.001$). Despite Clarke and Clarke's (1984) critique, Krieger has rightly stressed the observable relaxation response which results from therapeutic touch. This is supported by the complementary studies of Heidt (1979) of the effect of touch on state anxiety, Keller and Bzderk (1986) on tension headache, and Boguslawski (1980) on pain relief.

Nurses at Oxford nursing development unit have received basic instruction in therapeutic touch and massage. Empirical observation has so far confirmed Krieger's 'relaxation response'. providing comfort and aiding sleep and pain control. Massage, amongst other holistic practices is also currently being used on a cardiology ward at Charing Cross Hospital London by Sister Maggie Hill (Holmes, 1986).

Skill in the selection, combination, application and evaluation of therapeutic nursing measures is a crucial one requiring careful study. This will come with more extensive use of such measures and the recording of such observations as to their effect on patients. All approaches are arbitrarily classified here; however, they are unified by their therapeutic potential for the recipient of nursing care.

NURSING BEDS AT BURFORD (BNDU) AND OXFORD NURSING DEVELOPMENT UNITS (ONDU)

Three nursing beds are established at Burford nursing development unit, funded by the Sainsbury family trust. Beeson ward in the Radcliffe Infirmary, Oxford, is the home of the Oxford nursing development unit, where 16 nursing beds are provided. Nursing beds cater for patients in a rehabilitation setting for those in a post-acute phase of their illness. Such patients, while continuing to need intensive nursing have a significantly less intensive need for medical care.

The origins of BNDU and ONDU lie originally at the Loeb Center for Nursing in New York. Other influences are the nursing centres at Rush and Rochester Universities in the United States (Pearson, 1983). Both British units were established by Dr Alan Pearson: Burford in 1981, and Oxford in November 1985.

Beeson ward was set up by money provided by the Sainsbury family trust with building and service support from Oxfordshire Health Authority. It is the setting for the main nursing bed study piloted at Burford (see Table 4.1).

The units are perhaps most closely based upon Pearson's (1983) vision of a 'clinical nursing unit' which provides professional nursing as the chief therapy. It strives to become a centre for exploring and developing nursing practice with an accompanying emphasis on clinical education and research. The unit is committed to overcoming the divergence that exists between nursing theory and practice which, argues Miller (1985b), continues today. ONDU is the first of its kind in this country, being based in a large hospital.

An important step towards establishing an effective clinical unit was to make the nursing philosophy explicit from the beginning. A specific nursing model was chosen and discussed to aid this process. Roper, Logan and Tierney's (1980) model was used because of the nurses' familiarity with its use, a wish to use a British model initially, and the need to get the unit operational immediately. The units philosophy also incorporates much of Hall's concept of nursing, described above (pp. 75–77).

Admission to the unit depends on referrals from the acute hospitals in Oxford. The admission criteria and procedure have been explained (see Table 4.1). Although at present there are restrictions to the types of patients admitted because of the study design, it it envisaged that in the future any patient with a primary need for nursing, who is out of 'biological crisis', would be admitted.

At the end of 1985 a decision was made to open six of the unit's beds to patients in any medical category whose main need was for nursing. Study patients continued to get preference.

THE FUTURE OF NURSING BEDS

Nurses must strive to ensure that those people in need of their services receive the best they can offer. Questions of the best use of resources are paramount at a time of a continuous process of rationalisation in the NHS. The favourable indications of the effectiveness of nursing beds in meeting patients' needs at lower costs is an important enough issue to warrant continuation of the ONDU study to completion. It is only through experimentation and careful study that we are more likely to find more effective ways of organising the nursing service.

Fear of the loss of 'medical beds' is likely to provoke vested interest and pockets of resistance to such developments. Perhaps the proposed non-partisan general manager will prove his worth here in working for the best public service.

Whether the trials with nursing beds are given a fair run or not nurses must continue to make it known when they are aware of health needs that they can strive to meet.

Mahler (1985) of WHO has said: 'nurses will become resources to people rather than resources to physicians'. As they become increasingly adept at this perhaps the potential effectiveness of nursing in meeting basic health needs will be realised by society. Diers (1981) has recognised this: 'Nurses will be placed in positions which make demands on their skills and their personal competence that are extraordinary and not matched in any previous period in our history.'

REFERENCES

Alfano, G. (1985) 'Whom Do You Care For?'. *Nursing Practice*, 1(1), 28–31.

Baly, M. (1975) *Professional Responsibility*. (Wiley and Sons, Chichester).

Baly, M. (1980) *Nursing and Social Change*. (Heinemann, London).

Bellaby, P. and Oribabor, P. (1980) 'The history of the present contradiction and struggle in nursing', in Davis, C. (ed.) *Rewriting Nursing History*. (Macmillan, London).
Berger, P. and Luckmann, T. (1971) *The Social Construction of Reality*. (Penguin, Harmondsworth).
Boguslawski, M. (1980) 'Therapeutic Touch: A Facilitator of Pain Relief'. *Topics in Clinical Nursing*, 2(1), 27–37.
Boore, J. (1978) *A Prescription for Recovery*. (RCN, London).
Bradshaw, S. (1986) Personal communication with Senior Nurse (Geriatrics) Radcliffe Infirmary, Oxford, 17 June and 1 July.
Briggs Report (1972) *DHSS Report of the Committee on Nursing*. (HMSO, London).
Campbell, A. (1984) *Moderated Love: A Theology of Professional Care*. (SPCK, London).
Capra, F. (1982) *The Turning Point: Science, Society and the Rising Culture*. (Fontana, London).
Carpenter, M. (1977) 'The New Managerialism and Professionalism in Nursing', in Stacey, M. *Health and the Division of Labour*. (Croom Helm, London).
Cartwright, A. (1964) *Human Relations and Hospital Care*. Institute of Community Studies. (Routledge and Kegan Paul, London).
Clarke, P. and Clarke, M. (1984) 'Therapeutic Touch: Is There a Scientific Basis for Practice'. *Nursing Research*, 33(1), 37–41.
Cormack, D. (1985) (ed.) *Geriatric Nursing — A Conceptual Approach*, p. 93. (Blackwell, Oxford).
Daily Telegraph (1986). Article, 13 May.
Davis, B. (1984) *Preoperative Information Giving: An Implementation Study. Report to SHHD*. (NRU Edinburgh, core programme project).
Davis, B. (1985) 'The Clinical Effect of Interpersonal Skills: The Implementation of Preoperative Information Giving', in Kagan, C. (ed.) *Interpersonal Skills in Nursing: Research and Applications*. (Croom Helm, London).
DHSS (1976) *Prevention and Health: Everybody's Business*. (HMSO, London).
DHSS (1978a) *Physically Disabled People Living at Home: A Study of Numbers and Needs. Report on health and social subjects*, 13. (HMSO, London).
DHSS (1978b) *A Happier Old Age*. (HMSO, London).
DHSS (1981) *Social Trends (OPCS)*. (HMSO, London).
DHSS (1985a) *Experimental NHS Nursing Homes for the Elderly*. (HMSO, London).
DHSS (1985b) *Hospital In-Patient Enquiry (OPCS)*. Series MB4 No. 22. (HMSO, London).
Diers, D. (1981) 'Clinical and Political Issues in Nursing Practice', in Hockey, L. (ed.) *Current Issues in Nursing*, p. 79. (Churchill Livingstone, Edinburgh).
Doyal, L. (1979) *The Political Economy of Health*. (Pluto Press, London).
Dubos, R. (1959) *Mirage of Health: Utopian Progress and Biological*

Change. (Anchor Books, New York).

Field, D. (1976) 'The Social Definition of Illness', in Tuckett, D. (ed.) *An Introduction to Medical Sociology*. (Tavistock, London).

Franklin, B. (1974) *Patient Anxiety on Admission to Hospital*. RCN Research Series. (RCN, London).

Friedson, E. (1975) *The Profession of Medicine*. (Dodds, Mead, New York).

Garraway, W.M., Akhtar, A.J., Prescott, R.J. and Hockey, L. (1980) 'Management of Acute Stroke in the Elderly: Preliminary Results of a Controlled Trial'. *British Medical Journal*, 280, 1040–1043.

Gingell, J. (1985) 'Nursing Practice and Accountability', in Sykes, M. (ed.) *Licensed to Practice: The Role of the Staff Nurse*. (Baillière Tindall, London).

Hall, L. (1964) 'Nursing, What Is It?' Address to the Virginia State Nurses Association, 12 September 1958, *Canadian Nurse*, 60, 150–154.

Hall, L. (1969) 'The Loeb Center for Nursing and Rehabilitation, Montefiore Hospital and Medical Center, Bronx, New York'. *International Journal of Nursing Studies*, 6, 81, 88.

Hall, L., Alfons, G., Rifkin, E. and Levine, H. (1975) 'Final Report: Longitudinal Effects of an Experimental Nursing Process', unpublished, p. 6. (Loeb Center for Nursing, New York).

Hayward, J. (1975) *Information, A Prescription Against Pain*. RCN Research Series. (RCN, London).

Heidt, P. (1979) 'An Investigation into the Effects of Therapeutic Touch on Anxiety in Hospitalised Patients', *unpublished PhD thesis*, New York University.

Henderson, V. (1960) *Basic Principles of Nursing Care*. (ICN, Geneva).

Hill, J. (1985) 'Nursing Clinics for Arthritics'. *Nursing Times*, 18 September.

Hockey, L. (1978) 'The Future Nurse: Selection and Training; Autonomy; Should Her Health Care Role be Modified for Future Patient Demands', *Journal of Advanced Nursing*, 3, 571–582.

Holmes, P. (1986) 'Fringe Benefits'. *Nursing Times*, 82(22), 20 and 22.

ICN (International Council of Nurses) (1973) *International Code of Nursing Ethics*. (ICN, Geneva).

Illich, I. (1976) *Limits to Medicine: Medical Nemesis — the Expropriation of Health*. (Penguin, Harmondsworth).

Jacox, A. (1978) 'Professionalisation of Nurses', in Chaska, N. (ed.) *The Nursing Profession; Views Through the Mist*. (McGraw-Hill, New York).

Jourard, S. (1971) *The Transparent Self*. (Van Nostrand, Princetown, New Jersey).

Kalisch, B.J. (1979) 'Of Half Gods and Mortals: Aesculapian Authority', in Turner, G. and Mapa, J. (eds) *Humanising Hospital Care*. (McGraw-Hill Ryerson Ltd, Toronto).

Keller, E. and Bzdeik, V. (1986) 'Effects of Therapeutic Touch on Tension Headache'. *Nursing Research*, 35(2), 101–106.

Kennedy, I. (1981) *The Unmasking of Medicine*. (George Allen and

Unwin, London).

Kinlein, M. and Young, K. (1977) 'Independent Nurse Practitioner: Concept of Practice'. *Nurse Practitioner*, 2(6), 10–12.

Kitson, A. (1984) 'Steps Toward the Identification and Development of Nursing Therapeutic Functions in the Care of Hospitalized Elderly', *unpublished PhD thesis*, University of Ulster, Coleraine.

Kitson, A. (1985) 'Educating for Quality'. *Senior Nurse*, 3(4), 11–16.

Krieger, D. (1981) *Foundations for Holistic Health Practices*, pp. 4, 138. (J.B. Lippincott Co., Philadelphia).

LeMay, A. (1986) 'A Discussion of Methods Being Used to Establish the Nature and Frequency of Nurse–Patient Touch and its Relationship to the Wellbeing of Elderly Patients'. Paper delivered at 1986 RCN Research Society Conference. Reading University (unpublished).

Leininger, M. (1985) *Care: The Essence of Nursing and Health*, p. 3. (Thorofare, New Jersey).

Levi, P. (1985) 'Hospital Life can be Just What the Patient Orders'. *Daily Telegraph*, 6 November, 14–15.

Luker, K.A. (1982) *Evaluating Health Visiting Practice*. (RCN, London).

Macauley, C. and Anderson, A. (1974) 'The Nurse as Primary Therapist in the Management of the Patient with a Stroke'. *Cardiovascular Nursing*, 10, 7–10.

McFarlane, J. (1980) *Essays on Nursing*. Kings Fund Project Paper. (Kings Fund Centre, London).

MacGuire, J. (1980) *The Expanded Role of the Nurse*. (Kings Fund Centre, London).

Mahler, H. (1985) 'Nurses Lead the Way', *WHO Features*, no. 97.

Mapa, J. and Turner, G.P. (1979) *Humanizing Hospital Care*. (McGraw-Hill Ryerson, Toronto).

Marram, G. Schlegel, M. and Bens, E. (1974) *Primary Nursing: A Model for Individualised Care*. (C.V. Mosby, St Louis).

McKeown, T. (1976) *The Role of Medicine: Dream, Mirage or Nemesis*. (Nuffield Provincial Hospitals Trust, London).

Merrison Report (1979) *Royal Commission on the National Health Service*. Cmnd 7615. (HMSO, London).

Miller, A. (1985a) 'A Study of the Dependency of Elderly Patients in Wards Using Different Methods of Nursing Care'. *Age and Ageing*, 14, 132–138.

Miller, A. (1985b) 'The Relationship Between Nursing Theory and Nursing Practice'. *Journal of Advanced Nursing*, 10, 417–424.

Mitchell, J. (1984) 'Is Nursing any Business of Doctors? — A Simple Guide to the Nursing Process'. *British Medical Journal*, 283, 216–219.

Morgan, D. (1972) 'The Future Expanded Role of the Nurse'. *Canadian Nurse*, May, 75–80.

Naisbitt, J. (1984) *Megatrends: 10 New Directions Transforming Our Lives*. (Futura, London).

Neugarten, B.L., Havighirst, R.J. and Tobin, S.S. (1961) 'The Measurement of Life Satisfaction'. *Journal of Gerontology*, 16,

134–143.

Nightingale, F. (1859) *Notes on Nursing* (1980 edn). (Churchill Livingstone, Edinburgh).

Norris, C.M. (1970) 'Direct Access to the Patient'. *American Journal of Nursing*, 70, 1006–1010.

Orem, D. (1980) *Nursing; Concepts of Practice*. (McGraw-Hill, New York).

Pattie, A.H. (1981) 'A Survey Version of the Clifton Assessment Procedures for the Elderly (CAPE)'. *British Journal of Clinical Psychology*, 20, 173–178.

Pattie, A.H. and Gilleard, C. (1975) 'A Brief Psychogeriatric Assessment Schedule: Validation against Psychiatric Diagnosis and Discharge from Hospital'. *British Journal of Psychiatry*, 127, 489–493.

Pearson, A. (1983) *The Clinical Nursing Unit*. (Heinemann, London).

Pearson, A. (1985a) 'The Effects of Introducing New Norms into a Nursing Unit and an Analysis of the Process of Change', *unpublished PhD thesis*, University of London.

Pearson, A. (1985b) 'The Effect of Intensive Nursing on Patient Outcome', Study Proposal, Oxford Nursing Development Unit (unpublished).

Peplau, H. (1952) *Interpersonal Relations in Nursing*. (Putnam, New York).

Peplau, H. (1960) 'Talking with Patients'. *American Journal of Nursing*, 60(7), 964–966.

Pembrey, S. (1979) 'Vision of the Future'. *Nursing Mirror*, 30 August.

Phaneuf, M. (1976) *The Nursing Audit*. (Appleton-Century-Crofts, New York).

Prophit, P. (1986) 'Developing a Philosophy of Nursing: Academic Exercise or Practical Prerequisite for an Effective Nursing Service'. Seminar given at ONDU, Oxford, 4 February (unpublished).

Raphael, W. (1969) *Patients and their Hospitals*. (King Edward Fund, London).

RCN (1976) *RCN Code of Professional Conduct — A Discussion Document: Part III, Responsibility for Professional Document Standards*. (RCN, London).

RCN (1981) *Towards Standards*. (RCN, London).

Revans, R.W. (1964) *Standards for Morale: Cause and Effect in Hospitals*, Nuffield Provincial Hospital Trust. (Oxford University Press, Oxford).

Rogers, C. (1951) *Client Centred Therapy*. (Constable, London).

Rogers, M. (1972) 'Nursing: To Be or Not To Be'. *Nursing Outlook*, 20, 42–46.

Roper, N., Logan, W. and Tierney, A. (1980) *Elements of Nursing*. (Churchill Livingstone, Edinburgh).

Rowden, R. (1984) 'Doctors Can Work with the Nursing Process; A Reply to Professor Mitchell'. *British Medical Journal*, 288, 219–221.

Sackett, D. *et al.* (1977) 'The Role of the Nurse in Primary Health Care', Scientific Publication, no. 348. (The Organisation, Washington DC).

Schlotfeldt, R. (1972) 'This I Believe. Nursing is Health Care'. *Nursing Outlook*, 230, 245–246.

Skeet, M. (1970) *Home from Hospital*. (The Dan Mason Nursing Research Committee, London).

Stein, I. (1978) 'The Doctor–Nurse Game', in Dingwall, R. and McIntosh, J. (eds). *Readings in the Sociology of Nursing*. (Churchill Livingstone, Edinburgh).

Stevens, B. (1979) *Nursing Theory: Analysis, Application and Evaluation*. (Little Brown, Boston).

Telford, M. (1985) 'The Law and Nursing', in Sykes, M. (ed.) *Licensed to Practice: The Role of the Staff Nurse*. (Baillière Tindall, London).

Thomstad, B. (1975) 'Changing the Rules of the Doctor–Nurse Game', *Nursing Outlook*, 23, 422–427.

Tierney, A. (1984) 'A Response to Professor Mitchell's, A Simple Guide to the Nursing Process'. *British Medical Journal*, 288, 835–838.

Titmuss, R. (1958) 'The Hospital and Its Patients', in *Essays on the Welfare State*. (Allen and Unwin, London).

Travelbee, J. (1966) *Interpersonal Aspects of Nursing*, p. 19. (F.A. Davis, Philadelphia).

Veitch, A. (1986) 'BMA's Wounding Verdict on Rival Healers', and editorial 'Herbal Tea and No Sympathy'. *The Guardian*, 13 May 1986.

Versluysen, M. (1980) 'Woman Healers in English History', in Davis, C. (ed.) *Rewriting Nursing History*. (Macmillan, London).

Wade, B., Sawyer, L. and Bell, J. (1983) *Dependency with Dignity: Different Care Provision for the Elderly*. Occasional Papers in Social Administration, 68. (NCVO, Bedford Square Press, London).

Wandelt, M. and Ager, J. (1974) *The Quality of Patient Care Scale*. (Appleton-Century-Crofts, New York).

Weinberg, R., Liljestraud, J. and Moroe, S. (1983) 'Inpatient Management by a Nurse Practitioner: Effectiveness in an Rehabilitation Setting'. *Archives of Physical Medicine and Rehabilitation*, 64, 588–590.

Wilson-Barnett, J. (1978) 'Patients' Emotional Response to Barium X-rays'. *Journal of Advanced Nursing*, 3, 37–45.

Wilson-Barnett, J. (1984) *Key Functions in Nursing*. (RCN, London).

Wilson-Barnett, J. and Fordham, M. (1982) *Recovery from Illness*. (J. Wiley, Chichester).

Wilson-Barnett, J. and Osborne, J. (1983) 'Studies Evaluating Patient Teaching Implications for Practice'. *International Journal of Nursing Studies*, 20(1), 33–44.

5

Therapeutic Nursing

Plaxy-Anita Muetzel

INTRODUCTION

Nursing is most often perceived as an activity that supports the therapy of others, rather than being a therapy in itself.

The nursing development units at Burford and Oxford, however, see nursing as an activity with enormous potential for healing. The crucial determinant of whether nursing is therapeutic or not is the quality of the relationship between nurse and patient. The power of nursing to promote healing lies, we believe, in this therapeutic relationship.

THE THERAPEUTIC RELATIONSHIP

> Hopefully nursing practitioners will soon learn that nursing is a special case of loving.
>
> (Jourard, 1971)

The concept of the therapeutic relationship is not new and is apparently clear in its meaning — it sounds like the kind of helping, caring, nurturing togetherness, the desire for which brings thousands of candidates to nursing school interviews every year with the 'I-want-to-work-with-people' motivation. This togetherness is further defined by the candidate and young student in 'doing' words, and by a retired nurse (Mrs O'Keefe) interviewed by Maggs (1983): 'She cannot escape being turned into a competent nurse for the reason that with 30 or 40 beds in a ward and only three pairs of hands to attend them, she must always be nursing.'

It has indeed long been taught and examined as nursing knowledge and activities that shadow medical knowledge and activities. Even the term 'therapy' — last redefined in 1933! — has been adopted from this sphere, where it denotes (*Oxford English Dictionary*, 1933): 'The medical treatment of disease; curative medical treatment.' If, as suggested by McMahon (1986), nursing is a therapy in its own right, it must itself redefine therapy, its object and objectives. 'Therapy' suggests a deliverer and a recipient of treatment, but in the context of holism a therapeutic relationship should not only cater for 'the whole patient' but also 'the whole nurse'!

Central to the process of nursing, identified quite correctly if unclearly by eager candidates, is the patient–nurse relationship. At Oxford nursing development unit (ONDU) our conception of the relationship as therapeutic is suggestive of a purposeful, supportive and healing association between two persons that is *inter*active and holistic and further definable in 'being' words. It is *this* togetherness and *these* words that are the subject of this chapter; but to proceed to this without consideration of the moral philosophy of entering into such a relationship at all, and the nursing philosophy of united belief and direction, is as inappropriate in theory as it is in practice.

THE NEED FOR A PHILOSOPHICAL BASIS

Moral philosophy is at root a personal concern for the individual practitioner, requiring the examination of his own self-concept and personal needs, and the solutions to questions about the nature of Man: his responsibilities, requirements and rights; the meaning of suffering, and the purpose and dynamics of change in persons and the environment; the demands and limitations of personal 'blind spots' (Murgatroyd, 1985); and job description, perceived role and those of time and resources. A spectrum of answers to conscious and unconscious contemplations and learning determines the *kind* of 'work-with-people' an individual chooses or is drawn to in the first place.

Reviews of helping *methods* (for example, that of the National Education Association (1961) cited in Combs, Avila and Purkey, 1971) have failed to identify ones that are 'right'. Fiedler (1950) even found that experienced therapists of different schools held opinions on the requirements of a therapeutic relationship closer to each other and to 'the man in the street' than did beginners in the *same* school. Combs, Avila and Purkey (1969) have shown that it is those in whom a philosophy is developed and conscious who are judged by their patients/clients to be 'effective helpers', irrespective of their school of thought. Altschul (1972) argues strongly that training in helping professions ought to be a time of guidance in the clarification of such issues, and there are many authors for whom a continuing process of supported development and awareness of personal meaning, motivation and limits to personal competence is a minimum condition justifying professional practice (Jourard, 1971; Marteau, 1974; Blackham, 1974; Burnett, 1974; Murgatroyd, 1985). I would add that it is a privileged opportunity!

A nursing philosophy as a prerequisite for effective clinical practice has also been begged of its practitioners (Prophit, 1986; Leininger, 1984). This may be a structure, adopted by the nursing team, such as the Rogerian conceptual model of unitary man (Rogers, 1970), one of the first to break through the tradition-bound view of nursing as an intrinsic part of allopathic medicine. Alternatively, or in addition, it may be the result of a pooling of the less directly personal aspects of the individual moral philosophies brought to the team. Both strategies provide a shared system of beliefs concerning:

- the value of persons;
- the meaning of illness and health (both semantic and symbolic) — see, for example, Sontag (1983), also D.H. Lawrence's poem 'The Ship of Death' (Erwin and Thompson, 1978);
- the aims of the process of interaction with 'the sick person' and intervention in 'the sickness'; and
- the interrelationship of 'the sick person', with particular reference to the role of the nurse.

This 'shared system of beliefs' does not require them to be the *same* — just shared! 'It is the rigidity of beliefs that separates us from others' (Krishnamurti, 1954). Krieger (1981) puts it thus: 'The success of a holistic health orientation rests upon the individual's ungrudging ability to deeply examine previous assumptions, values, goals and relationships, and to radically change his or her world-view.'

The state is dynamic, facilitating a growing and maturing of meaningful and conscious self-concepts and world concepts. As a consequence, self-actualisation goes hand-in-hand with an advanced degree of professionalisation of individuals and their team. Thus equipped, the registered nurse becomes the renaissance nurse Krieger envisages for whom: 'at the core of holistic health practice is a philosophy that must be lived. Renaissance nursing is not a 40 hour a week job, but rather a 24 hour day commitment' (Boyd, 1981).

THE CORE OF THE BURFORD AND OXFORD NURSING DEVELOPMENT UNITS' PHILOSOPHY

The units' philosophy has been expounded elsewhere as it relates to:

● the needs of the patient post-biological crisis;
● the concept of nursing beds;
● the application of primary nursing, the nursing process and nursing models.

Sobel (1979) and Nichols (1984) compare and contrast technical and controlling medicine, which concerns itself with the restoration of function to, or arrested deterioration of, physical systems, and caring and healing medicine which supplies supportive information, instruction and intervention at physical, psychological and social levels; this is usually to minimise the impact of illness, hospitalisation/social isolation, and treatment. Here 'medicine' refers not only to the practice of doctors, but to the 'systems' provided for 'sick people', historically and culturally. Hence, such a philosophy of caring applies equally to the unit in the absence of active medical intervention (the second point above), to the needs of patients on traditional medical and surgical wards before and during biological crisis (the first point above), to the practices of 'alternative' or 'complementary' medicines, and even to the rituals of 'primitive' shamanism (Krieger, 1981; Grossinger, 1980).

The differences between these environments and approaches lie in their precise conception of the nature and desirability of a shortfall from physical, psychological, spiritual or social perfection, leading to different definitions of health and illness, and hence the behaviour considered appropriate to effect change in the direction required; for some disciplines actually *maximise* the impact of symptoms as in homeopathy (Hahnemann, 1962), or in the psychotherapeutic working — *through* a crisis (Berke, 1979) — even ECT has its roots in the apparent therapeutic effect of naturally occurring seizures (Sagar, 1972)!

Indeed, as said before, a constellation of beliefs concerning the nature of illness and health may coexist within *one* environment, especially in the current climate of revolution and renaissance in western health care.

Those amongst ONDU staff are perhaps more varied — ranging between conventional and controversial extremes — than in other nursing teams! I use the word 'constellation' to suggest that this variety is in itself meaningful and illuminating through dialogue with each other and 'other' health practitioners.

What *is* common to and significant in so many disciplines is the close, consistent and holistic association between the person seeking help (which may or may not correspond to his *requiring* it judged by others of his or any other society) and the person available, chosen, and (possibly) trained to give help of a particular kind (the third point above). It is this security of a way of 'being' and 'being with' that facilitates change, whether this be the return to an old way of life, adaptation to new circumstances, or to dying. This is essentially a developmental requirement. A remarkable study comparing Ugandan and European infants attributed the significantly more rapid achievement of 'milestones' of the former group to the far greater degree of physical and psychological security afforded by the custom of carrying the child wrapped close to the mother's body from birth (Geber, 1958). This view — long-appreciated or taken for granted outside the traditional western therapeutic system — is enjoying ever-increasing recognition in many of the helping professions familiar to us (Combs, Avila and Purkey, 1971).

At ONDU, as in a variety of nursing settings today, primary nursing aims to provide such an association, and it is specifically the resources and dynamics unique to each patient–nurse relationship that, in this team, is central to the therapy whose aim is rehabilitation — the process of ordering demanded by the disorder created by biological crises and consequent treatment in the life of an individual.

Disorder or disease is largely characterised in western

medicine by the virtue of its abnormality and, therefore, its undesirability rather than its unpleasantness (Downie and Telfer, 1980) which is the primary perception and basic concern of the sufferer. Help is rarely sought for organic and symptom-atological pathology that is *not* unpleasant, or else is preferable to feared diagnosis and treatment. It is the *intolerable* unpleasant-ness — the unsightly skin rash or sore, the inconvenient incontinence or ingrowing toenail, the painful broken arm or ageing process — that brings a person to medical care, where subjective symptoms may or may not find sympathy and/or effective treatment. Whether or not either or both are supplied, unless the sufferer is referred for psychiatric assistance for a 'complaint' judged to be 'in the mind', the nurse is often the per-son of whom it is required to alleviate any residual, untreatable or 'hypochondriacal' physical and mental unpleasantness.

'Only pain *perceived* as curable is intolerable' (Illich, 1976) (my italics), and where pain, disfigurement, permanent infirmity or terminal conditions are at the heart of suffering, it is the nurses's unique, privileged and challenging role not only to provide the traditional tender loving care, but a very active stimulus and environment for psychological and spiritual change — a change in attitude that perceives unpleasantness in a new tolerable, accepting and creative light.

Downie and Telfer (1980) point out that: 'The old-fashioned or religious-sounding noun "healing" covers more of the ground required for the aim of medicine than our common modern word "health" .' Pietroni (1986) has proposed that 'the pursuit of health' can be seen as one of today's greatest sicknesses. Holistic health practice of healing is not immune to this sickness, and can easily be seduced by the goal of Whole Health. Wholeness *is* of itself. True holism should impose no conditions. Wholeness through healing is the uniqueness and completeness of the person — quite literally, warts and all!

This discussion argues for the necessity and contribution to practice of moral and nursing philosophies by demonstrating the relevance of the 'being' of caring for the practitioner, the team and the recipient. Kitson (1986) has appealed for a methodology to validate the hitherto intangible and elusive qualities of caring. 'Intuition and experience' are daily used to justify action, but since a hit-and-miss attitude is morally and professionally indefensible where persons of value are con-cerned, this mystique of the nurse demands to be brought to consciousness and clarity, and a place in the research base and methodology of practice. Once achieved, not only can its essence be communicated and taught but its influence may *inform* caring by providing guidelines for the selection of methods and a frame of reference for prescriptive choices for action and interaction, allowing nursing to be a truly 'creative effort' (Orem, 1980).

It is our belief in the nursing development units, inspired by the work of the Loeb Center (Hall, 1969; Hall *et al.*, 1975) that it is the 'therapeutic use of self' (Jourard, 1971; Travelbee, 1971), which *can* be calibrated and used predictably through a conscious philosophy, in the context of the relationship made possible by primary nursing; that is the primary tool.

THE OBJECT AND OBJECTIVES OF THERAPY

'This is a pervasive therapy — something that gets into the blood-stream, not a poultice applied locally' (client, in Rogers (1951), p. 93). In recent years awareness of the traditional allegiance of nursing to the 'medical model' has inspired the evolution of a number of 'nursing models', for example, Henderson (1960), Roper, Logan and Tierney (1980), Orem (1980), Reihl (1980), Roy (1980). The one adopted most widely in this country — as at BNDU and ONDU — has been that of Roper, focusing on the activities of daily living. The activities specified are functional and behavioural, and there is a grave potential danger of interpreting them and their associated problems as such. This merely results in the 'medical model' in a modern guise, and is particularly apt to happen in the absence of clear moral and nursing philosophies.

Where the philosophical basis of care is concerned with 'being' and 'a need for relationship for security and change', activities of daily living have the flavour of *ways* of daily *being* about them. All activities are significant only in relation to the *meaning* they have in themselves for a person (Frankl, 1963), and within that person's unique and evolving web of meanings, within which disability and disease are or become a significant, even creative *part* (Leitner, 1980). This has also been called self-actualisation (Maslow, 1962), the dynamic pattern of humanness (Progoff, 1963), the growth principle (Combs, Avila and Purkey, 1971), the process of becoming (Allport, 1955), dissonance reduction (Festinger, 1962), the search for self-fulfilment (Rogers, 1961), and self-consistency (Lecky, 1945). The philosopher J.S. Mill (1962) paints the following picture:

> Human nature is not a machine to be built after a model and set to do exactly the work prescribed for it, but a tree which requires to grow and develop on all sides according to the tendency of the inward forces which make it a living thing.

The ability to walk may mean the ability to get to the lavatory or to make a cup of tea to the housebound, or the necessity of fetching groceries once a week, or the joys of walking the dog twice a day or backpacking twice a year. Through enquiry the nurse may rapidly grasp the functional/behavioural needs of the patient and set the realistic goals demanded by the nursing process, and may prescribe and implement appropriate action. If, however, she fails to recognise the motivational factors present or absent, though the patient may resist (for people only learn that which is consistent with their meanings or relevant to problems as they are perceived) or else 'get better' in spite of her 'doing', there is a sense in which he remains a patient to his nurse and to himself, without uniqueness, opinion, dignity or value. Consider the truth of the word 'invalidity'? This is a state fostered particularly efficiently by the physical and emotional environment of institutions in which loss of privacy, freedom and individuality provide absolution from responsibility, and coercion to cooperate with those who 'know best'. It is sobering to think not only of hospitals in this light, but also, for example, of the education system, the army, and the nursing profession whose members are all at risk of suffering invalidity!

Combs, Avila and Purkey (1971) note that: 'Helping people to change their perceptions of themselves and the world requires a different kind of model from that required to change the physical body.' Where nurse and patient are not merely in association, but in a relationship whose nature is holistic and therapeutic, a confrontation and a sharing of meanings will occur (Macrae, 1981) in which both have the power to influence change and in which both are *vulnerable* to change! Wheelchair mobility may be no compensation per se for the amputee's collapse of meanings. He may withdraw into denial, or he may well 'get better' and be discharged home to the care of the community and artificial limb services. The opportunity for meaningful change and healing *beyond* the physical will, however, have been lost by the invalid and the nurse who perceived him as such.

RELATIONSHIP AS PARTNERSHIP, INTIMACY AND RECIPROCITY

Travelbee (1971) states: 'It is one of the tasks of the professional nurse to perceive and respond to the human being in "the patient" and to assist the ill human being in responding to the human being who is "the nurse".' He draws attention to five orientations that may characterise the patient–nurse interaction:

● automatic
● helpful
● involuntary
● minimal
● inconsistent

It is interesting to consider how these attitudes on the part of the nurse — those we observe and ourselves if we are honest! — have different implications for 'doing':

● automatic doing   'usually'   — action in accordance with ward routine
● helpful doing   'ought'   — action in accordance with a desire for satisfaction or reward
● involuntary doing 'must'   — action in accordance with perceived expectations of others
● minimal doing   'only'   — action in accordance with apathy, or bitterness towards colleagues or 'the system'
● inconsistent doing 'like'   — action in accordance with absence of vulnerability

The 'human-to-human interaction' is on the other hand, 'a mutually significant experience' — a recipe for authenticity leading to self-actualisation for both, in accordance with the meeting of personal philosophies.

The components of the relationship that validate both individuals may be identified as partnership, intimacy and reciprocity. Partnership is another way of describing that working association between two parties (who are not necessarily equals) in a joint enterprise, and which implies gains for both. Patients and nurses have always been partners. It is the balance of power and equality that has recently come into question. Intimacy is a closeness at physical, psychological and spiritual levels which suggests a sense of communion between persons that is meaningful and valuing to and of those concerned. After many years of contributions to literature (see, for example, Peplau, 1969; Jourard, 1971; Travelbee, 1971) the value of intimacy is gradually gaining respectability in theory, if only reluctant recognition in practice. Sadly, students (and indeed qualified nurses) are still criticised today by those who 'know best' for getting 'too involved with the patient'. The concept of reciprocity is more threatening still for it suggests that the nurse too can be receiver not only of information and cooperation, but also of support and care!

Figure 5.1

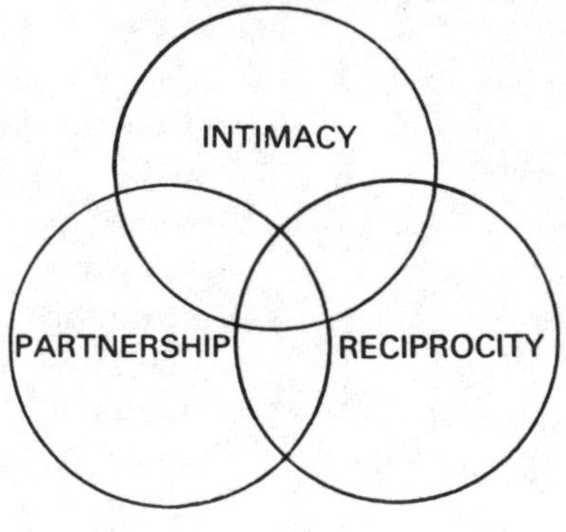

There are large areas of overlap between these components (Figure 5.1), but for the sake of discussion and clarity the components of the therapeutic relationship may be polarised somewhat according to the parameters shown in Figure 5.2. This permits separation and identification of the specific

Figure 5.2

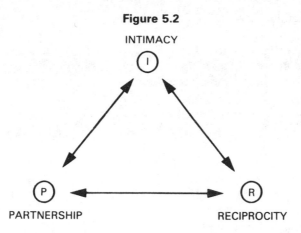

qualities that characterise areas of overlap and the substance of the encounter that flourishes in their presence (Figure 5.3).

Figure 5.3

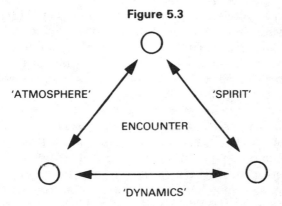

Although reductionist (!), it is helpful to break down this expanded structure into its constituent pairs, to examine its dimensions more closely. This, it is hoped, will demonstrate the manner in which the 'atmosphere' of the encounter (that is, intimacy and partnership ➞ the attitudes we *have*), the 'dynamics' of the encounter (that is, partnership and reciprocity ➞ the things we *do*) and the 'spirit' of the encounter (that is, reciprocity and intimacy ➞ the way we *are*) unite in a 'whole-istic' therapeutic relationship.

Partnership ←— —→ **intimacy**

Considering first the dimensions spanning the more accepted parameters of partnership and intimacy, the qualities of security and freedom are most prominent.

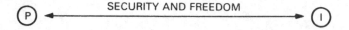

Many authors have dwelt on these qualities far more comprehensively than is appropriate here, where our intention is to focus on their relevance to 'the human being in "the patient" . . . and the human being who is "the nurse" '.

Security

The value of security as a developmental prerequisite from the beginning of life has already been touched upon. For the infant, whose experience is primarily sensual, physical security is fundamental, direct and relatively uncomplicated. Throughout life 'growth is movement into the unknown-unpredictable . . . into the known-predictable . . . Each such assimilation and adaptation to the unknown increases the scope of the known . . . increases the ability to move into more unknowns' (Chilton-Pearce, 1979).

Eventually the unknown-unpredictables encompass emotional, intellectual and existential anxieties that challenge a matrix of bio-psycho-socio-spiritual known-predictables (that is, the personal philosophy). It is at times of crisis that gentle oscillations in this rhythm reach extremes that may be over-whelming, and when the security required for assimilation and adaptation is less tangible, less direct, and highly complex in its demands of the professional helper. If the crisis of physical trauma or disorder is associated causally and/or consequentially with disease throughout a personal matrix, it is the unique role of the nurse, as 'a generalist among specialists' (Lahiff, 1981) to provide an environment that is emotionally as well as physically secure.

The complexity of providing security for another that is conducive to change lies in the empathy and unconditional positive regard described by Rogers (1951) — in the degree of acceptance of another (that is, another's matrix) required of the helper, and hence the degree of self-awareness in the helper (that is, development of personal matrix) from which the other self is to be distinguished and beside which it is to be valued. Koestler (1949) describes empathy as 'mental resonance'. Carkhuff and Benzon (1982) elaborate on the 'atmosphere' of security, presenting the following factors as those identified by recipients in the counselling situation as particularly helpful:

● increased awareness
● recognition of similarity
● core conditions perceived (that is, empathy, warmth, genuineness)
● expressiveness
● open communication
● warmth (helper is himself and not playing a part)
● ventilation (in a safe and neutral atmosphere).

Freedom

That the nurse with clear personal and professional philosophies is thus able to distinguish more readily between her own perceptions and those of her patient, *and* able to convey this, is perhaps stating the obvious. It is, however, precisely this developed and communicable subjectivity, in a profession keen to develop objective and 'scientific' standards, that has great implications for her capacity not only to predict behaviour accurately — a characteristic of empathy (Travelbee, 1971) — but also to resist judgement of the causes and manipulation of the consequences of another's predicament. Moral judgement, if negative, renders 'help' patronising, devoid of compassion, and hence mechanical; if positive, 'help' becomes protective, devoid of respect and literally *self*-indulgent, through over-identification. According to Davitz and Davitz (1981) such judgements result in the inappropriate empathy whose origins are present in the expectations and attitudes of early training, and whose development is often haphazard and negative leading to an unspoken 'professional subculture' — a sort of unconscious nursing philosophy.

Jourard (1971) cautions against 'specialisation' of the nurse in patients ('white people', 'normal people', 'neuters') who do not challenge or offend the values of her own personal matrix and who therefore elicit an unhelpful sympathy, while the rest are condemned and invalid as persons (because they are black,

101

psychiatrically or psychologically disturbed, or are men who make passes!). The ability to avoid directive manipulation of another's direction of change arises out of: 'the assumption that the human organism is predictable and, provided it has the proper conditions for freedom, can be counted on to move towards desirable ends' (Combs, Avila and Purkey, 1971). These conditions are *belief* — rather than assumption — not only in the moral *right* of another to choice and control, but also in his trustworthiness to make meaningful and adaptive changes. This very point was illustrated impressively in a health service setting by the so-called Peckham experiment (Pearse and Williamson, 1938) and in a nutritional health education context (Lewin *et al.*, 1942).

Even when apparently meaningless and maladaptive to the nurse's perceptions, 'desirable ends' *may* include the choice of the sick role (whether 'genuinely', 'hypochondriacally', or 'psychosomatically'; Wilson-Barnett, 1979; Siegel, 1986). Whether, when and how interference *is* justifiable is yet another moral issue for the nurse (Downie and Telfer, 1980).

It is one of the responsibilities, then, of the nurse as a catalyst for change to establish and maintain this curious and difficult tension between security and freedom. The patient, whose self-concept is so easily dominated by a sense of inadequacy through enforced dependence in the first place (Sermat and Smythe, 1973), cannot help but respond to a genuine affirmation of the validity and authenticity of his past sufferings, present condition and fears for the future with an echo that relinquishes denial and resistance to help and change (Nichols, 1984). Hilgard (1978) cites the comforting and liberating experience from the pain of terminal cancer under the therapeutically induced hypnotic state where: 'patients can experience for themselves that they are more complex and complete than that aspect that is involved with the pain'.

The facilitating effect of an atmosphere of this nature was powerfully demonstrated to the participants in the recent Dartington Conference: Re-Visioning Illness. The Conference Director urged this collection of self-confessed 'wounded healers' from a very broad spectrum of disciplines to accept and love the 'dark, messy bits' in themselves and in others (Kidel, 1986). Once these shadows assumed equal status with the 'sparkling, interesting bits', a sense of completeness and confidence was born of the safety to be and the liberty to become. This is surely the essence of healing, for 'health authorities' are not areas or regions, or bodies of practitioners and administrators, but authority belongs to nurse and patient alike, to the individual whose right and in whose power it is (or to whose power it is to be restored) to direct the passage from cradle to grave. Health authority is conferred through the special atmosphere of the working association of partnership between human beings in the health care setting and the honest confrontation of intimacy.

Partnership ◄── ──► reciprocity

The dimension spanning the parameters of partnership and reciprocity can be aptly described thus: 'the challenge for nurses and health education is to help the older person feel like a more powerful participant in the process of health care' (Salveson, 1981). This is, of course, particularly applicable to ONDU patients, but the call for the ingredients of communication, contract and control are equally appropriate in very many health care settings. With imagination, the challenge may be interpreted with even the most unlikely candidates!

$$\text{(P)} \xleftarrow{\hspace{1cm}} \text{CONTROL + CONTRACT + COMMUNICATION} \xrightarrow{\hspace{1cm}} \text{(R)}$$

Contract

It is a significant feature of the patient–nurse encounter, that the latter so often *assumes* consent to this association of the former, whose participation, in whatever sense –– active or passive –– may be quite involuntary, although necessitated through circumstance. Sierra-Franco (1978) points out that health practitioners and patients differ in the degree to which their roles are chosen or forced upon them; in other words, the nurse chooses her profession, whereas the patient is a victim of accident or sickness. Nevertheless, it has been noted earlier that 'choice' of the sick role *does* occur and it should be added that 'the human being who is "the nurse"' may be the victim of a role in which she is perceived!' It seems, however, that definition and consciousness of role and the advantages of control and power –– and therefore responsibility for them –– lie clearly with the nurse, in contrast to the disorder of the enforced sick role, where 'extinction is feared less than the process that brings about the progressive dissolution of the things that have been considered to be the act of living' (Osis, 1961).

It is, therefore, one of the responsibilities of the nurse to redress the balance, using initial assets to initiate purposeful communication and to establish a contract of *shared* power, control and responsibilities that is acceptable to both and which clarifies the relationship of needs presented and resources available — 'the complimentarity of agency' (Orem, 1980).

The process of making a contract is another way of achieving a sense of security through converting unknown-unpredictables to known-predictables, this time in a more factual and practical way. Information in the medical setting as a 'prescription against pain' of all kinds is well documented (Hayward, 1975). Murgatroyd (1985) — referring to the counselling situation lists the following ingredients of the helping relationship about which the person to be helped may have expectations and anxieties.

- gender of helper
- social background/ understanding of helper
- confidence/competence of helper
- duration of relationship

- amount and times of contact

- helper's style of working
- ethics of relationship, for example, confidentiality
- specific purposes of relationship
- conditions for termination of relationship
- contact with helper outside and beyond relationship

It is the responsibility of the nurse to confirm, correct or compromise with these by providing not only new information, but also the sensitive affirmation and flexibility — with a recognition of personal fallibility — that permits the patient to draft the contract too.

Control
Herein lies a sensitive issue — that of the degree of directiveness beneficial or permissible in the helping relationship. Lippitt and White (1952) conducted an experimental study of styles of helping relationships which they identified as:

- authoritarian

● *laissez-faire*
● democratic

but which, in practice, were often found to overlap, providing a continuum of ill-defined and therefore unpredictable and insecure environments. They observed how democracy in particular could easily be replaced by autocracy, which can be *imposed* through creating dependence or the perception or attitude of dependence. On the other hand democracy needs to *grow* through fostered independence and self-direction, which is where the paradox of assisted self-determination arises — in the counselling situation: 'the person who asks for help because he wishes to control his own destiny' (Packer, 1974).

Traditionally, nurses (amongst other blue-collar workers including hospital personnel), faithful to the medical model, have tended to be very directive (that is authoritative and socially restrictive in their care; see Cohen and Struening, 1963) and this has indeed been welcomed and encouraged to a large extent by the patients who derived security in the knowledge that 'nurse knows best'. It is impossible to dictate from model or theory or philosophy of nursing how an individual practitioner is to conduct any one relationship. There are so many factors on which the extent of the directive element depends, such as once again the personal philosophy of the nurse — her needs for control, power and satisfaction and her perception of the needs and rights of another; and the personal philosophy of the patient — his self-concept in the light of his present condition and his perception of his abilities, strengths, needs and rights; and the demands and restrictions of the environment in which the encounter takes place, for example, accident service, paediatric or terminal care ward, surgical or community setting.

Packer (1974) suggests that:

> an influence which is acceptable to the client and which does not bind him to inappropriate resolutions of his personal task can validly be directive in form and structure in so far as it may leave the client with freedom of choice when he comes to draw his conclusions.

The way in which this is to be achieved is a question that necessitates conscientious consideration by the individual practitioner in the context of close team-consultation, ensuring a conscious and consistent approach to the individual patient.

Communication

Its implementation demands a high degree of proficiency in communication skills of the nurse, about which a great deal has percolated in recent years into the professional literature from the theoretical realms of psychology and the practical sphere of counselling. Nevertheless, this remains an area of infamous complacency, and O'Brien (1978) cautions that: 'communication is difficult precisely because it is assumed to be easy'! She describes it as a process involving coding of the unique perceptions of the sender, and decoding of these by the receiver to match and compare the information received with his own unique perceptions. Information thus 'converted' and 'comprehended' then needs to be checked against that *intended*, so that understanding is a process of evolution, rather than an escalation and subsequent collapse of assumptions.

Combs, Avila and Purkey (1971) point out that most interactions are dialogues with both parties seeking personal enhancement, and that the helping relationship requires one temporarily to set aside his own needs. Since, however, both nurse and patient as human beings and as roles *require* personal enhancement — in a nutshell, the former as 'professional satisfaction', the latter as 'comfort' — the nurse whose responsibility it is to conduct effective communication is quite justified in assisting both parties in achieving this. The unknown territory of reciprocity is approached here, which challenges the traditional long-suffering altruism of the nurse. If we are indeed to love others as we love ourselves, self-definition and self-enhancement for *both* then: nurse as facilitator (Hall, 1969) — guarantor of care (Nichols, 1984), model and teacher (Smith, 1981; Watts and Hardy, 1985), agent of (social) reality (Packer, 1974); actualiser of health potential (Krieger, 1981); and patient as achiever (Hall, 1969)—gradually resuming responsibility for self (O'Brien, 1978), responsible for successful self-defined outcome (Hollender, 1958), must be components of contract and natural consequences of communication in the context of the whole relationship.

Reciprocity ← — → intimacy

'Being there' is that intangible and paradoxically difficult and

106

very simple essence of the dimension of reciprocity and intimacy. It is simple because it is in the desire for closeness of the philanthropic vocation 'to help people', difficult because a closeness that is mutually beneficial in a therapeutic relationship requires mature confrontation by the nurse, in this situation, of the vulnerability of her own humanness.

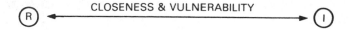

Wilson-Barnett (1979) points out the paucity of research evidence on how patients are helped with all kinds of distress, and yet an undisputed common denominator in circumstantial evidence proves to be the mere presence of a nurse and her willingness to listen: 'of all the life-saving equipment that helped me, the presence of another human being was the most essential' (Jeffries, 1964). Nursing research has indeed lagged far behind theoretical proposal — preferring more scientific pursuits than this — for the qualities of human-to-human relatedness and vulnerability (Travelbee, 1971); closeness (Peplau, 1969), and self-disclosure (Jourard, 1971) have been represented in the literature for some time.

Closeness

Peplau (1969) describes closeness as 'not so much a matter of being "closer" to the person who is ill, but rather one of being "closer to the truth" of that person's current dilemma', which is the basis for effective help where the knowhow to use such understanding exists. She appeals for a mature and conscious emotional involvement to aid the more detached clinical process of observation and analysis in the development of understanding.

Muetzel (1980) showed, in a comparison of psychiatric nurses and psychology students at either end of their respective courses, how it is the latter who achieve a hypothetical closeness, becoming more accepting towards 'abnormal' stereotypes and optimistic of their capacity for self-responsibility and change. Sadly the group of nurses demonstrated increased caution, hostility, feelings of helplessness, and even unwillingness to become involved with or care for such physical, psychological and social 'misfits' over the course of their training. Extrapolation from such results is hazardous but the implications of this for individual nurses, and the profession, let alone for the patients, give cause for concern.

A hypothetical closeness is easily developed in an academic environment, and through the discussion of facts and concepts, beliefs and feelings, practitioners from such a background may indeed be at an advantage once a *real* patient is encountered. Personal reactions to relationships may then be informed by the knowledge of study and the knowing of introspection. It has long been assumed and boasted that nurses learn 'by experience', but such experience without supervision and guidance from those more experienced, and peer support within a team is, as the study above suggests, prone to tragically negative consequences for all concerned.

Vulnerability

It was Menzies (1960) who first systematically observed and documented thoroughly the defence mechanisms common in nursing practice that provide *apparent* protection against the anxieties of involvement with patients. These serve to detach the nurse from her feelings, to assist her denial of personal vulnerability, and to depersonalise the patient in her perceptions. Menzies proposed, however, that avoidance of anxiety, guilt, doubt etc. avoids their confrontation and hence the reassurance and satisfaction of their resolution. This leads to all manner of secondary anxieties and a phenomenal waste of energy in maintaining defences.

It is obviously not only the nurse who loses out but also the patient. Viscott (1976) notes that: 'people with no vulnerability have no sensitivity. They also cannot respond to another's feeling because they have no access to their own feelings.' Travelbee (1971) speaks of the access to the sufferings of another in which caring becomes an 'act of courage', and where suffering as a spiritual experience may become meaningful and enriching for both.

There is here no wish to suggest that a human-to-human encounter in the spirit of closeness and vulnerability on the part of the nurse should encroach on the privacy and modesty of the patient or anyone else. They do not equate with familiarity, and the degree of self-disclosure possible and appropriate is another issue for philosophies and contracts.

It is suggested, however, that there is in this particular

dimension of the therapeutic relationship something that allows the nurse to benefit from the association by receiving from the patient in the most direct sense, for it is often the case that it is not so much assistance as *permission* that is required by 'the ill human being in responding to the human being who is "the nurse"'. The 'being there' for another is required at this level of relationship, where shared tears and tissues are in themselves meaningful and meet suffering in a place which is, in the first instance, quite inaccessible to techniques and technologies. Siegel (1986) hopes, tongue in cheek, that love 'once it is scientific, it will be accepted'. Shunned thus far by nursing research, it is these areas of relationship that remain a challenge to nursing theory and to the practice of a holistic therapy of nursing.

THEORY MEETS PRACTICE

This chapter has repeatedly drawn attention to the uniqueness of the individual, and the importance for patient and nurse of the latter clarifying the uniqueness of herself as a human being that she brings to a working association between them. For different patients in different settings it will be appropriate that this association develops to different degrees according to the qualities described — as well as others identified or favoured by the reader — providing an acceptable relationship holding the potential for therapeutic change for both. It is the responsibility of the 'human being who is "the nurse"' to determine the kind of environment, 'type' of patient, and style of working compatible with her skills and needs — both personal and professional.

The nurses working in the Burford and Oxford nursing development units represent a range of personalities, backgrounds and ambitions, sharing, so it sometimes seems, little more than the belief that the basis of caring and healing is not so much what the nurse *does* to or for the patient, but that a close and consistent relationship between two people — rather than roles — provides the vital ingredient and that this is rarely possible to such an extent under the restrictions of other settings, much less capitalised on (for example, in student–nurse/patient associations).

It follows, therefore, that without a strict formula Burford and Oxford nursing development units relationships are as varied as anywhere else — indeed the *aim* is greater variety. Through professionally facilitated staff support meetings, and less structured caring interactions between nurses, stereotyped defensive attitudes and behaviour patterns are gradually identified and exorcised.

The substance of the encounter is represented here by a sample of nursing issues and activities in the context of partnership, intimacy and reciprocity as they have been discussed (Figure 5.4).

Figure 5.4 Nursing issues and activities in the context of partnership, intimacy and reciprocity.

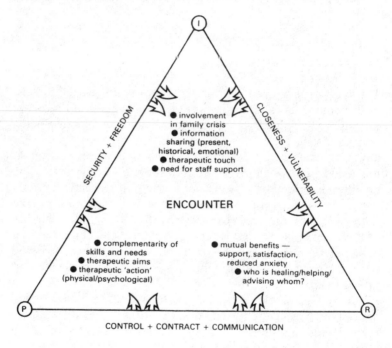

● involvement
in family crisis
● information
sharing (present,
historical, emotional)
● therapeutic touch
● need for staff support

SECURITY + FREEDOM

CLOSENESS + VULNERABILITY

ENCOUNTER

● complementarity of
skills and needs
● therapeutic aims
● therapeutic 'action'
(physical/psychological)

● mutual benefits —
support, satisfaction,
reduced anxiety
● who is healing/helping/
advising whom?

CONTROL + CONTRACT + COMMUNICATION

Apparent polarisation is again only for the sake of clarity and suggests no more than, for example, that the complementarity of skills and needs is characterised by the genesis of the association in the first place, although change and resolution of that association may depend heavily on intimate and reciprocal caring; that the practice of therapeutic touch is principally

110

characterised by intimacy, though may bear witness also to partnership and reciprocity; that rehabilitation is not so much a question of dependence converted to independence, but of healing interdependence characterised by reciprocity though clearly supported by an intimate working partnership.

The process of developing relationships in the nursing development units might be likened to a masked ball at which hosts and guests gradually reveal their true identities, to find they much prefer each other's natural and varied complexions and expressions to the rigid, if highly decorative, masks.

The nurse, as host, has responsibility for welcoming the guests, for initiating events and interactions that create and maintain the desired atmosphere, and for ensuring that the guest is sent on his way home satiated, cheered, with pleasant memories and pleased to have come! The patient, as guest, is in this case invited to participate in a research project exploring a new style of nursing environment. Having accepted, he arrives, 'in costume', only to find that his hosts in fact are not! That the nurses are wearing their own clothes is the first and most obvious observation. Rather than formal announcements and introductions, nurses offer Christian names — a small number identifying themselves as personal hosts — and ask for a preferred name in return, altogether very informal. Nurses and patients are perched together on unmade beds, discussing care plans and charts over cups of coffee in a ward that even after 9.30 in the morning still has a 'homey' look about it! Mealtimes are a sharing not only of food but of thoughts, happenings, worries, jokes and music between guests and hosts alike.

An oriental philosopher observed that 'to know a man is not to know a man but to know his melody'. In the units the nurse/hosts initiate the unmasking of themselves and their patient/guests at a pace and in ways according to the qualities brought to each unique relationship. For the former, it may be through the mature and honest expression of anger or frustration over 'unreasonable' behaviour in the latter. For the latter it may be the permission to keep a lifelong daily routine — *and* the ability to respond to that permission, which can be difficult, even for the most mildly institutionalised, who expect the nurse to arrange the pillows, or bring tea round for everyone at once at their *own* convenience!

A joint unmasking occurs in such shared experiences as massage, whether to relieve pain, constipation, tension or insomnia, when conversations, or simply a silent communion that can be equally revealing and enriching, become free. The physical benefit alone for each human being may be that *both* relax, and where the patient falls asleep the night nurse is left to combat soothed and altered consciousness with caffeine!

Intimate and reciprocal sharing at many levels makes partnership in caring and healing a more concrete reality in the units. When nurse/host and patient/guest truly recognise and appreciate each other in the wholeness of the genuine and valued human being beneath the masks conferred by role and expectation, each can take their partner by the hand and in harmony take steps in a shared direction.

REFERENCES

Allport, G.W. (1955) *Becoming: Basic Considerations for a Psychology of Personality*. (Yale University Press, New Haven, Connecticut).

Altschul, A.T. (1972) *Patient/Nurse Interaction: A Study of Interaction Patterns in Acute Psychiatric Wards*. (Churchill Livingstone, Edinburgh).

Berke, J.H. (1979) *I Haven't Had to Go Mad Here*. (Penguin, Harmondsworth).

Blackham, H.J. (ed.) (1974) *Ethical Standards in Counselling*. (Bedford Square Press of the National Council of Social Service, London).

Blattner, B. (1981) *Holistic Nursing*. (Prentice Hall, Englewood Cliffs, New Jersey).

Boyd, N.E. (1981) 'We Are One: The Renaissance Nurse as Neighbour', in Krieger, D. (ed.) *Foundations for Holistic Health Practices*. (J.B. Lippincott Co., Philadelphia).

Burnett, J. (1974) 'Values and Assumptions in the Psychodynamic Content of Counselling', in Blackham, H.J. (ed.) *Ethical Standards in Counselling*. (Bedford Square Press of the National Council of Social Service, London).

Carkhuff, R. and Benzon, B. (1982) *Intentional Changes — A Fresh Approach to Helping People Change*. (Follett Publishing, Chicago).

Chilton-Pearce, J. (1979) *Magical Child*. (Paladin, London).

Cohen, J. and Struening, E.L. (1963) 'Opinions About Mental Illness: Mental Hospital Occupational Profiles and Profile Clusters'. *Psychological Reports*, 12(1), 111–124.

Combs, A.W., Avila D.L. and Purkey W.W. (1969) *Florida Studies in the Helping Professions*. University of Florida Social Science Monograph no. 37. (University of Florida Press, Gainesville, Florida).

Combs, A.W., Avila, D.L. and Purkey, W.W. (1971) *Helping Relationships: Basic Concepts for The Helping Profession*. (Allyn and Bacon Inc., Newton, Massachusetts).

Coutts, L.C. and Hardy, L.K. (1985) *Teaching for Health — the Nurse as Health Educator*. (Churchill Livingstone, Edinburgh).

Davitz, J.R. and Davitz, L.L. (1981) *Inferences of Patient's Pain and Psychological Distress*. (Springer Publishing Co., New York).

Downie, R.S. and Telfer, E. (1980) *Caring and Curing*. (Methuen, London).

Enelow, A. and McKinney-Adler, L. (1972) 'Basic Interviewing', in Enelow, A.J. and Swisher, S.N. (eds) *Interviewing and Patient Care*. (Oxford University Press, Oxford).

Erwin, D.W. and Thompson, E. (1978) 'ECT in Schizophrenia: a study in Eosobiotic Impressions'. In Brady, J.P. and Brodie, H.K.H. (eds) *Controversy in Psychiatry*. (W.B. Saunders, Philadelphia).

Festinger, L. (1962) 'Cognitive Dissonance'. *Scientific American*, 207, 93–107.

Fiedler, F.E. (1950) 'A Comparison of Therapeutic Relationships in Psychoanalytic, Non-directive and Adlerian Therapies'. *Journal of Consulting Psychology*, 14, 436–445.

Frankl, V. (1963) *Man's Search for Meaning: An Introduction to Logotherapy*. (Beacon, Boston).

Geber, M. (1958) 'The Psychomotor Development of African Children in the 1st Year and the Influence of Maternal Behaviour'. *Journal of Social Psychology*, 47, 185–195.

Grossinger, R. (1980) *Planet Medicine — from Stone Age Shamanism to Post-industrial Healing*. (Shambhala, Boulder, Colorado and London).

Hahnemann, S. (1962) *The Organon of Medicine*, 6th edn, translated by William Boericke MD. (Roysingh, Calcutta).

Hall, L. (1969) 'The Loeb Center for Nursing and Rehabilitation, Montefiore Hospital and Medical Center, Bronx NY'. *International Journal of Nursing Studies*, 6, 81.

Hall, L., Alfano, G., Rifkin, E. and Levine, H. (1975) *Final Report: Longitudinal Effects of an Experimental Nursing Process*, unpublished. (Loeb Center for Nursing, New York).

Hayward, J. (1975) *Information — A Prescription Against Pain*. RCN Research Series. (RCN, London).

Henderson, V. (1960) *Basic Principles of Nursing Care*. (ICN, Geneva).

Hilgard, E. (1978) *Divided Consciousness*. (John Wiley, New York).

Hollender, M.H. (1958) *The Psychology of Medical Practice*. (W.B. Saunders, Philadelphia).

Illich, I. (1976) *Limits to Medicine: Medical Nemesis: The Expropriation of Health*. (Penguin, Harmondsworth).

Jeffries, J. (1964) 'The Best Healing Device'. *American Journal of Nursing*, 64(9), 77.

Jourard, S. (1971) *The Transparent Self*. (Van Nostrand, Princeton, New Jersey).

Kidel, M. (1986) Unpublished Opening Address to Dartington Hall Conference on 'Re-Visioning Illness', 2 April.

Kitson, A.L. (1984) 'Steps toward the identification and development of nursing therapeutic functions in the care of hospitalized elderly'. *Unpublished PhD thesis*, University of Ulster, Coleraine.

Kitson, A.L. (1986) 'In praise of stout hearts and gut reactions', unpublished address to ONDU Seminar, 23 April.

Koestler, A. (1949) *Insight and Outlook*. (Macmillan, New York).

Krieger, D. (1981) *Foundations for Holistic Health Practices*. (J.B. Lippincott Co., Philadelphia).

Krishnamurti, J. (1954) *The First and Last Freedom*. (Harper and Row, New York).

Lahiff, M.E. (1981) *Hard to Help Families*. (HM and M, Aylesbury).

Lecky, P. (1945) *Self Consistency: A Theory of Personality*. (Island Press, New York).

Leininger, M.M. (1985) *Care: The Essence of Nursing and Health*. (Thorofare, New Jersey).

Leitner, I. (1980) Random article, in Hommes, U. (ed.) *Es Liegt an uns: Gesprache auf der Suche nach Sinn*. (Herder, Freiburg in Breisgan).

Lewin, K. *et al.* (1942) *The Relative Effectiveness of a Lecture Method and a Method of Group Decision for Changing Food Habits*. Mimeographed Report. (National Research Council, Washington DC).

Lippitt, R. and White, R.K. (1952) 'An Experimental Study of Leadership and Group Life', in Swanson, G.E., Newcomb, T.M. and Hartley, E.L. (eds) *Readings in Social Psychology* (rev. edn). (Henry Holt, New York).

Macrae, J.A. (1981) 'Listening: An Essay on the Nature of Holistic Assessment', in Krieger, D. *Foundations for Holistic Health Practices*. (J.B. Lippincott, Philadelphia).

Maggs, C. (1983) *The Origins of General Nursing*. (Croom Helm, London).

Marteau, L. (1974) 'The Counselling Relationship', in Blackham, H.J. *Ethical Standards in Counselling*. (Bedford Square Press of the National Council of Social Service, London).

Maslow, A.H. (1962) *Toward a Psychology of Being*. (Van Nostrand, Princeton, New Jersey).

McMahon, R.A. (1986) 'Nursing as a Therapy'. *The Professional Nurse*, July.

Menzies, I.E.P. (1960) 'A Case Study in the Functioning of Social Systems as a Defence against Anxiety'. *Human Relations*, 13, 95–121.

Mill, J.S. (1962) 'On Liberty', in Warnock, M. (ed.) *Utilitarianism*, Chap. 3. (Collins, London).

Muetzel, P.-A. (1980) 'An evaluation of the feelings, attitudes and beliefs of (1st and 3rd year) experimental psychology students and (1st and 2nd year) psychiatric nursing students towards the mentally ill and other stigmatised groups', *unpublished BSc thesis in experimental psychology*, Sussex University.

Murgatroyd, S. (1985) *Counselling and Helping*. Psychology in Action. (British Psychological Society and Methuen, London).

National Education Assocation (1961) Report in Combs, A.W., Avila,

D.L. and Purkey, W.W. (eds) *Helping Relationships: Basic Concepts for the Helping Professions.* (Allyn and Bacon, Newton, Massachusetts).

Nichols, K.A. (1984) *Psychological Care in Physical Illness.* (Croom Helm/The Charles Press, London).

O'Brien, M.J. (1978) *Communications and Relationships in Nursing.* (C.V. Mosby, St Louis).

Orem, D. (1980) *Nursing: Concepts of Practice.* (McGraw-Hill, New York).

Osis, K. (1961) *Deathbed Observations of Physicians and Nurses.* (Parapsychological Foundation, New York).

Oxford English Dictionary (1933) (Oxford University Press, Oxford).

Packer, A. (1974) 'The Directive Element in Counselling', in Blackham, H.J. *Ethical Standards in Counselling.* (Bedford Square Press of the National Council of Social Service, London).

Pearse, I.H. and Williamson, G. Scott (1938) *Biologists in Search of Material.* (Faber and Faber, London).

Peplau, H.E. (1969) 'Professional Closeness'. *Nursing Forum,* 8(4), 342–360.

Pietroni, P. (1986) 'Health and Illness — A Balance of Opposites', unpublished address to seminar at Dartington Hall Conference on 'Revisioning Illness', 3 April.

Progoff, J. (1963) *The Symbolic and the Real.* (McGraw-Hill, New York).

Prophit, P. (1986) 'Developing a Philosophy of Nursing: Academic Exercise or Practical Prerequisite for an Effective Nursing Service'. Seminar given at ONDU, Oxford, 4 February, unpublished.

Reihl, J.P. (1980) 'The Reihl Interaction Model', in Reihl, J.P. and Roy, C. (eds) *Conceptual Models for Nursing Practice.* (Appleton-Century-Crofts, Norwalk, Connecticut).

Rogers, C. (1951) *Client Centred Therapy.* (Constable, London).

Rogers, C.R. (1961) *On Becoming a Person.* (Houghton Mifflin, Boston).

Rogers, M.E. (1970) *An introduction to the Theoretical Basis of Nursing.* (F.A. Davis, Philadelphia).

Roper, N., Logan, W. and Tierney, A. (1980) *Elements of Nursing.* (Churchill Livingstone, Edinburgh).

Roy, C. (1980) 'The Roy Adaptation Model', in Reihl, J.P. and Roy, C. (eds) *Conceptual Models for Nursing Practice.* (Appleton-Century-Crofts, Norwalk, Connecticut).

Sagar, K. (ed.) (1972) *D.H. Lawrence: Selected Poems.* (Penguin, Harmondsworth).

Salveson, C. (1981) 'Holistic Health for the Elders', in Krieger, O. *Foundations for Holistic Health Practices.* (J.B. Lippincot, Philadelphia).

Sermat, V. and Smythe, M. (1973) 'Content Analysis of Verbal Communication in the Development of a Relationship — Conditions Influencing Self-disclosure'. *Journal of Personal Social Psychology,* 26, 332–346.

Siegel, B.S. (1986) 'Love Medicine'. *New Age Journal,* April.

Sierra-Franco, M.H. (1978) *Therapeutic Communication in Nursing.* (McGraw-Hill Inc., New York).

Smith, J.P. (1981) *Nursing Science in Nursing Practice.* (Butterworths, London).

Sobel, D. (1979) *Ways of Health: Holistic Approaches to Ancient and Contemporary Medicine.* (Harcourt, Brace, Jovanovich, New York).

Sontag, S. (1983) *Illness as Metaphor.* (Penguin, Harmondsworth).

Travelbee, J. (1971) *Interpersonal Aspects of Nursing*, 2nd edn. (F.A. Davis, Philadelphia).

Viscott, D. (1976) *The Language of Feelings.* (Arbor House, New York).

Wilde-Mayerson, E. (1976) *Putting the Ill at Ease.* (Harper and Row Inc., New York).

Wilson-Barnett, J. (1979) *Stress in Hospital: Patients' Psychological Reactions to Illness and Health Care.* (Churchill Livingstone, Edinburgh).

6

Nursing and Intimate Physical Care — the Key to Therapeutic Nursing

Angela Wharton and Alan Pearson

As previous chapters have highlighted, the nursing units are based on the fundamental belief that nursing is essentially a therapeutic activity which involves the reaching out of one person — the nurse — to another person who needs assistance, teaching, or support — the person who is nursed — in a practical way.

In inpatient care, this frequently involves help with very intimate or private activities. The nurse is seen as the only health worker who can legitimately become involved in very intimate touch, as in toileting and bathing. Simple though such tasks may be in physical terms, being involved in such encounters can offer the opportunity to the nurse of becoming closer to the patient or client, and this growing closeness can be used in a therapeutic way. Regarding intimate physical care as 'basic nursing' or 'common sense' means that it may be delegated to the untrained and thus opportunity to develop closeness may well be lost. As previous chapters show, *all* direct nursing care in the units is carried out by registered nurses, because these apparently simple acts involved in intimate physical care are seen as the key to therapeutic nursing, human touch can be used as a powerful vehicle for comforting and healing, and nurses are trained to develop touch further through the use of therapeutic massage.

THERAPEUTIC TOUCH

Hall *et al.* (1975) describe how intimate physical touch so commonly an inherent part of delivering nursing care, can lead

117

to closeness between nurse to patient, and argue that this closeness can be used therapeutically. Whilst nurses can easily become blasé about intimate activities such as bathing patients, or become skilled at distancing themselves from such acts as cleaning incontinent patients or performing mouth toilets, the units' nurses are encouraged to value the opportunity to get close to people through such seemingly 'basic' yet potentially embarrassing encounters. It appears to be a relatively easy assignment to strip someone naked, immerse them in a bath of water, and clean the skin with soap, if this is viewed as a practical, mechanical task. It is, however, extremely skilled and complex if viewed as an intensely intimate and personal activity. When carried out as a simple physical task, it can lead to an embarrassed, unhappy and belittled patient, and a bored, dissatisfied nurse. When viewed as an opportunity for close-ness, however, it can lead to the shared identification of previously unrealised or undetected problems, the growth of an intimate understanding between nurse and patient. On employment, all nurses in the unit are introduced to this philosophy and attend an ongoing course on therapeutic touch.

THE NURSING TEAM'S APPROACH TO THE USE OF TOUCH IN THE UNITS

The theoretical background

The everyday use of intimate physical touch is seen in the unit as an area of complexity with its own conceptual framework. This form of non-verbal communication has been described by Barrett (1972) as the first and most effective method of communicating. Locsin (1985) suggests that people share themselves with other people, and at the same time gain knowledge of others. In nursing, touch 'says I care; being touched means I am worthy of care' (Ernst and Shaw, 1980).

Although touch is valued and seen as therapeutic, the concept of 'personal space' is of importance in the use of touch; while many people do derive therapeutic benefit when nurses use touch sensitively, others resent it and see it as an invasion of their personal space. The cultural background, sex, age, and expectations of individuals influence their attitudes to being touched by others, and these all demand respect and sensitivity.

Two kinds of touch

Touch occurs in two main contexts in nursing: in the process of performing a procedure or giving intimate physical care; and deliberately in the course of conversation, counselling or teaching.

Procedural touch

This is by far the most common in nursing, and includes the touching of intimate parts of the body in activities such as bathing and toileting, as well as holding someone's hand while a painful procedure is being carried out, or their wrist when taking a pulse rate. It occurs out of necessity, in other words it is part of the procedure, and therefore is frequently ignored as an important part of non-verbal communication. However, if it is always acknowledged as an act of intimacy, this form of touch can give comfort.

Non-procedural touch

Although less used than procedural touch, this is very common in nursing. Nurses frequently touch patients when the procedure does not require it, or in general conversation. However, non-procedural touch is often routinised, and nurses have used it indiscriminately in a way they would never do to people they meet who are not patients. Consequently, this type of touch is often seen as the impersonal act of a nurse who does it to everyone, and is sometimes resented by those who dislike physical contact with strangers. If touch is used in this context in a planned way, and where permission is subtly negotiated so that patients who find it difficult to accept are given the opportunity to make this clear, it has enormous therapeutic potential.

Both procedural and non-procedural touch which is routinised, rough, and indiscriminate can be actively antitherapeutic, in that brusque or rough touch can impair relationships between the two people involved. While many writers on therapeutic touch suggest it has specific healing powers (Krieger (1975), for example, describing it as a process whereby an energy field surrounds the body), the unit nurses use touch as a purely empathic form of communication for comfort.

Valuing the use of touch in practice

Unit nurses are encouraged to use touch in a conscious and planned way, and to establish with the patient whether or not physical touch is acceptable to him or her. Those who make it clear that they do not like to be touched except where absolutely essential, have this preference respected, and it may, with the patient's permission, be incorporated into the care plan. Where this is not the case, some forms of planned touch can be incorporated into the care plan. For example, one unit patient shared her dread with her nurse of the daily dressings she needed to have on an open wound on the stump of an amputated limb. During the procedure, she 'tensed up', which made her back ache, and she 'felt like screaming'. It was finally agreed that another nurse would be asked to carry out the dressing, and the patient's own nurse would put her arms around the patient, enabling her to rest her head on her shoulder, while the nurse gently and lightly massaged the patient's back. This was incorporated into the plan of care. On evaluation after three days, the patient said she no longer dreaded the procedure, and felt that she could now cope with the dressing if her nurse just held her hand. More importantly, the nurse and patient had become much closer, and the patient openly expressed the strong feeling she now held that her nurse took her seriously and that she could be more open with her than she ever thought possible in hospital.

Because touch is highly valued, and its appropriate use is seen as a valuable nursing activity, it is used frequently and often commented upon by visitors to the unit.

MASSAGE

A logical extension of the use of touch is the incorporation of massage into nursing care. Just as touch is inherent in many nursing acts, massage too is a well-established nursing intervention. Its use, however, has lessened in the last 20 years. It has come to be seen as a rather basic skill, with no underlying principles, which can be carried out by anyone. Consequently, massage is undervalued in pain relief and insomnia. All unit nurses undertake a course in massage taught by a qualified, experienced masseur/masseuse, and regular monthly ongoing practical workshops on massage are conducted by a local qualified masseur/masseuse in the Oxford unit, voluntarily attended by nurses from both units.

THE NURSING TEAM'S APPROACH TO THE USE OF MASSAGE IN THE UNIT

The theoretical background

Massage, one of the oldest forms of comfort and healing, has until fairly recently become a lost art in nursing, taking second place to high technology interventions and the use of drugs. The unit's philosophy incorporates the belief that massage is an essential component of nursing, and an extremely effective nursing intervention for pain, sleeplessness, anxiety, stress, and for creating a feeling of wellbeing. It increases the blood supply to muscles and tissues, and relaxes and tones muscles. As well as its very real physical/physiological effects, like touch, it also helps to promote closeness between nurse and patient, and the positive benefits this has on the nurse–patient relationship can be used to therapeutic effect.

When used for pain relief, massage can be carried out anywhere on the body where pain is felt, as long as the nurse notes that: if pain is felt by the patient from the massage, then it is too vigorous; and massage of the spine is to be avoided. A variety of massages can be used for the resolution of stress, anxiety, and sleeplessness, and the aim for all of these problems is to induce relaxation and a feeling of wellbeing. All unit nurses are taught, through formal and practical teaching, to carry out massage of head and neck, scalp, hand, foot and full body. Some nurses attend further training to learn other massages, and some also train in reflexology. The six basic massages, however, are needed by all nurses, and the monthly 'top-up' sessions are provided in an attempt to ensure that these skills are maintained and developed. Grapeseed oil is usually used for massage, although some patients prefer to use their own body lotions.

121

Using and valuing massage in the units

Massage is seen in the units as a useful, everyday nursing intervention, and is used extensively. When a specific massage is thought to be indicated, the nurse negotiates with the patient to establish if it is acceptable, and the goals of the massage are agreed upon. The intervention is then incorporated into the plan of care. The most frequent nursing problems which are amenable to massage, and for which massage is prescribed are: pain in the shoulder, hands, knee, back, and foot (when medical assessment rules out suspicious cases); anxiety/ tenseness; inability to sleep.

Specific massages for specific problems vary according to patient need and preference, and the judgement of the nurse, but pain in the shoulder, hands, knees, and foot is usually treated by gentle kneading and massaging of the painful area and the surrounding skin using grapeseed oil, having warmed the hands first. In addition, painful feet are first soaked in warm water and dried thoroughly before massage. As well as gentle kneading, the nurse makes circles over the whole of the sole of the foot using the thumbs, and the sole of the foot is also stroked using the knuckles of one hand.

Back pain

For back pain, a back massage is carried out as follows:

- The patient lies on the abdomen, and the bed is pumped up to its highest position.
- After warming the hands and oil, the hands are placed on the back and left there for a few seconds before commencing massage to enable both nurse and patient to relax. Using the oil as lubricant, the massage is commenced beginning on the lower back and moving upwards slowly, using firm, definite strokes.
- When the neck is reached, the shoulder blades are gently kneaded.
- The sides of the patient are then massaged using long, downward strokes.
- The lower back is then massaged using the thumbs, and quick, short strokes away from the nurse towards the patient, keeping close to the spine.

● Finally, the whole back is kneaded starting at the shoulders and working down the back. The spine is not massaged heavily because it has little muscle coverage.

Anxiety, tenseness, sleeplessness

Anxiety, tenseness, and sleeplessness are usually treated by one of the following massages, or a combination of two or more: head and neck; foot; full body; back; scalp. Massage for the head and neck, and foot, have been found to be particularly useful for sleeplessness.

The use of massage by nurses has become highly valued, as a useful, non-invasive alternative to drugs and technological intervention. The use of night sedation in the units has fallen notably since the initiation of massage for sleeplessness; a number of patients have found massage more effective than analgesics for pain. Some of these patients suffering chronic pain for a number of years have been dependent on analgesics.

The use of massage in the units is not seen as an optional extra, or a trend to follow. It is highly valued as a nursing skill and this is reflected in the commitment to training of nurses through employing outside experts in massage. The specific massages are considered to be quite complex, and all nurses must be thoroughly trained to carry them out effectively. Training only some members of the nursing team would mean that massage could not be incorporated into care plans in an ongoing way. Similarly, the units' nurses believe that carrying out massage without expert training is of little therapeutic use.

CONCLUSIONS

Using the hands to comfort and heal is an ancient art, and is seen as an essential nursing skill in the nursing units, and as a logical extension of the nurse's role in giving intimate physical care. Therapeutic touch and massage are well within the competence of the nurse if taught thoroughly, are beneficial to patients in themselves, and contribute towards the development of a close nurse–patient relationship. The complex, therapeutic role of both primary nurse and associate nurse, rooted in close relationships and an environment for healing and growth, hinges, we believe, on the hands of the nurse being used therapeutically in giving direct care.

REFERENCES

Barrett, K. (1972) 'A Survey of the Current Utilization of Touch'. *International Journal of Nursing*, 9, 195–209.
Ernst, P. and Shaw, J. (1980) 'Touching is not Taboo'. *Geriatric Nursing*, September.
Hall, L.E., Alfano, G.J., Rivkin, M. and Levine, H.S. (1975) *Longitudinal Effects of an Experimental Nursing Process*. (Loeb Center for Nursing, New York).
Krieger, D. (1975) 'Therapeutic Touch'. *American Journal of Nursing*, May.
Locsin, A.C. (1984) 'The Concept of Touch'. *Philippine Journal of Nursing*, 54(4), 114–23, 140.

7

Developing Clinical Nursing

Alan Pearson

INTRODUCTION

The purpose of this final chapter is to summarise the key principles of primary nursing and nursing beds, as adapted and applied in the Burford and Oxford nursing development units, and to compare them with current trends and developments in the wider world of nursing in general. The chapter therefore consists of reviewing the contents of previous chapters, and then applying this to current nursing ideology by means of a general discussion.

The Burford and Oxford nursing development units were originally established to develop clinical nursing in order to help patients, increase cost effectiveness, and improve the job satisfaction of clinical nurses. The work is essentially in its infancy, but already after four years important lessons have been learnt and fundamental principles have been established. The preceding chapters have attempted to describe briefly how nursing practice is organised, how nursing beds are run, and how the process of caregiving is based on therapeutic relationships and the therapeutic use of touch and massage. The theoretical and philosophical underpinning of these approaches has been discussed in depth. Within the units, nursing is seen as a therapy in itself, and is delivered by an all-registered nursing team with a high level of support from non-nurses who are accountable to nursing. The nursing team itself is composed of primary nurses and associate nurses, who are enabled to practise through the support of senior nurses who take a consultative role. In both units, patients are admitted primarily for nursing, and the patient's own nurse acts as keyworker in close collaboration with other members of the multidisciplinary clinical team. Nursing care focuses on the notion of nursing as a therapy, and incorporates the creation of a relaxed, open, and therapeutic environment and the creative use of touch. Nurses do not wear an institutional uniform, and they share meals with patients to make mealtimes a social occasion. Patients have access to their own case notes, and take their own medication.

Like the Loeb Center for Nursing in New York (Pearson, 1983), the style of nursing practised has many critics. Their major criticisms relate to costs, feasibility elsewhere, and the lack of evidence that the unit's philosophy has beneficial effects. More fundamental, however, is apparent resistance to radical change in health care by nurses and other health care professionals. Much of the unit's work bears a striking resemblance to proposals for change by nurse leaders throughout the world, and to the growing demands for a more individualised, human, and holistic approach to health care by consumer groups. A number of questions can be asked:

● Are the Oxfordshire units described in this book merely pipedreams of utopia, inappropriate for replication elsewhere?
● Are they luxurious and too expensive, or are they possible everywhere?
● Are they an elitist attempt by egotistical Oxford nurses to win praise, or are they a genuine attempt to put into action a vision of what some nurses believe nursing is all about?
● Are they an example of a trendy radical bandwagon, or do they really reflect the long-term aspirations of a growing number of nurses?

Obviously, the unit's staff identify with the positive sides of these either/or statements, and believe that much of the philosophy developed is the way forward in developing clinical nursing, and in its survival as an essential component of health care.

OVERVIEW OF THE KEY PRINCIPLES OF PRIMARY NURSING IN THE DEVELOPMENT UNITS

The units have attempted to be explicit in three major areas concerning nursing, namely: the nature of nursing, the management of care, and the management of nursing.

The nature of nursing

The units have reached explicit agreement within the multidisciplinary team that nursing is a therapeutic activity in itself which aims at helping people to feel better, and to use this to achieve as much independence as is possible for the patient. Patients are viewed as individuals who are 'whole persons', with a right to participate in decisions about their own lives and health. Nurses achieve successful nursing outcomes through the establishment of close relationships with their patients, and by using this closeness to therapeutic effect in a planned, systematic way, subject to continuous evaluation. These views of nursing and of the patient are discussed with all health care disciplines working in the unit, and are explored in joint training sessions using simulated patients (Pearson, Morris and Whitehouse, 1985). As a result of this, the environment is patient-oriented, and professional work revolves around the agreement that the nurse is the keyworker and coordinator of care.

While nursing is often seen as a support service to 'therapists' (for example, doctors, physiotherapists, occupational therapists etc.), in some areas it is seen as a therapy in itself in that nursing actually has a healing effect. Other disciplines serve to support nursing. In caring for the whole person, the nurse has expertise in giving physical, psychological and social care, but all interventions aimed at this provision of care are in essence social acts, and therefore warm, close human interaction is highly valued. Such sentiments and beliefs about the nature of nursing are often voiced generally in nursing, but applying them in reality has demanded a radically different approach to the management of care in the units.

The management of care

Based on explicit agreement on the nature of nursing, the management of care in the units is markedly different from many other inpatient settings. The atmosphere is deliberately informal: staff do not wear uniforms, furniture is less institutional in appearance, and there are no restrictions on visitors. Folding beds are provided to enable relatives and friends to stay overnight, and facilities for making hot drinks are provided in the ward areas. In the Oxford unit there is a bar stocked with both alcoholic and soft drinks, and this is to be provided in the Burford unit. The patient's day is governed by his/her own preference, and there is a policy that no patient will be wakened in a morning, except where there is a specific request for a morning call. Breakfast is served between 7.30 am and 11 am, and fixed mealtimes (that is, lunch and dinner) are social occasions where nurses and patients sit together at a table and are served from tureens. There are no 'lights out' restrictions, and the daily routine differs for each patient. Patients may be referred to the Oxford unit by consultants or ward sisters, and to the Burford unit by general practitioners, district nurses, health visitors, or relatives. Admission is always by unit nurse practitioners.

On admission, time is taken to establish a working relationship between nurse and patient, before completing a holistic nursing assessment and construction of a problem-oriented plan of care. Other members of the multidisciplinary team contribute to the plan of care, and thus only one type of record is used. This is therefore patient-centred, rather than being professional worker-centred where each discipline keeps a separate record. Patients are encouraged to be aware of the contents of this record, which is kept in a file at the bedside. They are also free to contribute to the record themselves if they wish to. Nurses are helped to learn how to build close, 'real' relationships, to use physical touch therapeutically, and to carry out massage (see Chapter 6). Nurses who wish to be trained in other non-invasive complementary therapies are encouraged and enabled to do so, and are free to incorporate these into care plans where appropriate. For example, one nurse practitioner uses reflexology in her care, and another uses *tai chi* (a form of disciplined movement allied to dance) in his. Self-care is encouraged, and patients are helped to take their own medications, carry out their own dressings, etc. when possible.

The management of care centres on the individual patient's needs, and a belief in informality in an environment that makes people feel good. An activity organiser programmes entertainment such as music, dance and drama performances in the sitting room areas. The focus of care is the *person*, and the medical diagnosis is seen as one component of the person, rather than vice versa. When patient problems are resolved, discharge is planned by the nurse, in close consultation with the multidisciplinary team. The majority of patients have the opportunity of a home assessment, with the occupational therapist and nurse in attendance, and members of other disciplines where appropriate. All patients have the opportunity of a home trial with the nurse. This is different from a home assessment, in that the latter aims at assessing capability and determining needs, whereas the former is simply an excursion home to help the patient reorientate, and to smooth the transition from hospital to home. In the Burford unit, district nursing and health visiting are a part of the unit, and these community nurses are closely involved in discharge planning. In the Oxford unit, community nurses are consulted about discharge plans by telephone or letter. On final discharge, the patient is given a card with his/her nurse's name and work telephone number so that he/she feels free, in the early post-discharge period, to consult the nurse when appropriate.

Just as the philosophy of nursing demands a change in the management of care, the latter demands a different approach from the staffing structure and management of the units.

The management of nursing

In order to deliver the style of care discussed in this book, staffing and lines of accountability have to be geared to individualised approaches rather than routines. All nursing in the units is given by registered nurses. Student nurses are always supernumerary, and the units run effectively in the absence of students. Registered nurses, with the necessary skills and a minimum of two year's post-registration experience in practice, are appointed as primary nurses, and function as independent nurse practitioners with direct accountability to patients. Each primary nurse carries a caseload of up to eight patients and is responsible on a 24 hour, seven day a week basis for assessing and planning care. While on duty, she is also responsible for giving planned care and evaluating it.

Each nurse practitioner has a team of registered nurses who act as associate nurses. The associate nurse is responsible for carrying out care planned by the primary nurse and patient, and for evaluating this care. Unit patients are often acutely ill, dependent, and have major rehabilitative needs. The ratio of one nurse to eight patients makes it essential that the nurse is free to spend all of her time on duty in the patient areas. Support staff of high level in the form of care assistants are provided to deal with both cleanliness of the environment, and setting up and clearing away equipment, testing urine etc., while the nurse herself deals with the patient.

Care assistants also assist the nurse when two people are needed, and help the patient as would a caring relative. Care assistants do not give direct nursing care: they do not perceive themselves as nurses, and they are not perceived as nurses by patients. Nurses in the unit also need to be freed as much as possible from administrative tasks. A team of ward coordinators provide a back-up administrative service, and act as a reference point for visitors, other disciplines and telephone enquiries. Nurses carry two way 'walkie-talkies', so that the coordinators can pass messages on to them, and nurses can speak to the coordinators without leaving the patient area. Both care assistants and coordinators, though non-nurses, are employed on the nursing budget and are directly accountable to the nurses on duty. The multidisciplinary team relate directly to the nurse responsible for caregiving, and there is therefore no hierarchy in the day-to-day working environment. Although the nurse practitioner is a higher clinical grade than the associate nurse, with greater responsibility inherent in the role, associate nurses work opposite their own practitioner, and both nurses, when on duty, are explicitly accountable for the total care of a named group of patients.

RELATING KEY PRINCIPLES TO CURRENT DEVELOPMENTS IN CLINICAL NURSING

The 'vision' of how nursing should be

The management and delivery of nursing in the units is strikingly close to current ideas being voiced in nursing, and to modern management trends. The units, in many ways, represent the practical reality of applying contemporary views in the real world.

130

The code of professional conduct for nurses, midwives, and health visitors in the United Kingdom (UKCC, 1983) points clearly towards the development of a structure which makes the caregiving nurse directly accountable to the receiver of care. Primary nursing is a practical and realistic attempt to orientate the management of patient care in line with this code of professional conduct. In the current debate on setting standards and assuring quality, emphasis is now being laid on the need to promote the concept of the accountable or independent practitioner of nursing, who has a clearly defined accountability for a caseload, and who is charged with giving holistic care in a systematic way. Reports on monitoring standards in nursing and on the nature of clinical nursing frequently argue strongly for a strengthening of the role of the clinical nurse, and for a career structure that will allow nurses to gain more status and financial reward, without having to give up direct patient care activities (Royal College of Nursing, 1979, 1981). Nursing literature from all over the world has been based on the assumption that nursing should be holistic, systematic, and delivered by autonomous, accountable practitioners. In essence, the nature of nursing care and its management in the development units is no more than a practical application of the wealth of theoretical exhortations presented to clinical nurses by nursing's elite. Nursing in the development units is therefore the contemporary ideology of nursing in action.

The United Kingdom Central Council for Nurses, Midwives and Health Visitors suggests in its *Project 2000* (UKCC, 1986) that the future of nursing lies in developing the role of the practitioner, and that education must centre on preparing those who wish to nurse for functioning in roles that equate with those of nurse practitioner/primary nurse. The report cites Pembrey's (1985) cutting observation of the current state of nursing practice: 'Sadly [the] proper initial practitioner role does not exist; it is split between 'assisting' (the role of the enrolled nurse) and 'managing' (the role of the registered nurse in reality) and nursing drops through the vacuum in the middle.'

The crucial demands in the report include the need for an all-registered nurse workforce, and for a new 'assistant' workforce of 'aides'. The registered nurse is seen, however, as being a more autonomous and accountable practitioner who views the recipient of nursing as a whole person. Although the UKCC, as the partly elected controlling body for nursing, can rightly be seen as one representative voice of nurses, great disagreement ensued on publication of the report. Many nurses (as well as other health care workers) saw the report's vision of the nurse of the future, and of the educational preparation seen as necessary to produce such practitioners, as unacceptable. While some objection may arise out of a desire to protect vested interests, the ideology of nursing which has been carefully nurtured for the whole of the 20th century does, in fact, oppose the ideas inherent in *Project 2000* and in the sort of nursing practised in the Burford and Oxford units.

The 'reality' of how nursing is

The basic ideology which has always driven nursing is the human desire to nurture — a very human desire, unconcerned with male or female, young or old — the basic desire to reach out and help someone to feel better, more comfortable, happier, or cared for. No matter where a modern day nurse works, or how many high-sounding jargonistic terms she or he may use, if asked to describe the basis of nursing, the idea of nurturing (if not the word) would be used. If she or he were pushed further and asked to elaborate on nursing as an organised occupation, very often the need for a caring nature in the nurse would be mentioned; the need for a sound training, or knowledge base, would be pointed out; and the need for professionalism would be strongly advocated. Thus, the basis of clinical nursing would revolve around a professional with the capacity to care, and the knowledge and skills to do so, actually nurturing others, and this philosophy underlies the work in the development units.

The very fact there are people who are sick, or who are unable to care for themselves in such a way as to maintain healthy living, gives rise to the need for others in society to meet their needs. From the beginning of civilisation, it has been instinctively known that nurturing is essential to human life. The bulk of this is carried out by the parents of children, and the spouse, offspring or friends of adults. If one can equate nurturing with caring, Kitson (1984) has identified the essential characteristics of the carer or nurturer:

● the desire to care

- the ability to care
- the knowledge to care
- the respect for the person to be nurtured or cared for.

When one or more of these characteristics is absent in an ordinary member of society who is in a position to care or nurture, then a need arises for society to provide a specialist worker — someone who has been armed with these characteristics by undergoing a form of professional training. In our society, this has led to the creation of professional nursing. Survival of the human race, therefore, is inextricably linked with the development of professional nursing.

The philosophy which is said to underlie nursing is very clearly presented in the nursing media: nursing is caring; it focuses on the person; it is highly skilled; it is essential to the provision of health care; it requires training; it is a profession; it is loved by its recipients; it focuses on one human being reaching out to another and helping in a practical way, because the nurse has been educated to do so.

The media and groundswell folklore tell us that nursing is skilled human helping on a grand scale; it is selfless and demands a true vocation.

What then, the reality? It is perfectly obvious to us all that this noble view is pie in the sky, and something that few of us can actually achieve. But it is, of course, perfectly possible to at least value it and try to aim towards it. Alas, modern nursing appears to have deserted its original ethos, and although the public pay lip service to it as a profession that is skilled and that upholds the nature of the person as the humaniser of our health care system, that same public simultaneously decries nursing as simple 'women's work', and fails to reward nurses in the same way as other professional groups. Robinson (1946) points out that:

Woman is an instinctive nurse, taught by mother nature. The nurse has always been a necessity; and thus lacked social status. In primitive time she was a slave, and in the civilised era a domestic. Overlooked in the plans of legislators, and forgotten in the curricula of pedagogues, she was left without protection and remained without education. She was not an artisan who could obtain the help of a hereditary guide; there was no Hanseatic League for nurses. Drawn from the nameless and numberless army of poverty, the nurse worked as a menial and obeyed as a servant. Denied the dignity of a trade, and devoid of professional ethics, she could not rise above the degradation of her environment. It never occurred to the Aristotles of the past that it would be safer for the public welfare if nurses were educated instead of lawyers. The untrained nurse is as old as the human race: the trained nurse is a recent discovery. The distinction between the two is a sharp commentary on the follies and prejudices of mankind.

I would suggest that the follies and prejudices of society and nurses themselves, who are products of their own society, continue. 'Basic' nursing is devalued and denied by us as nurses, and the society in which we live, because of our ambivalence towards nursing which, on the one hand, worships high technology, and on the other sees caring as unskilled intuition inherent in woman.

Theoretical ideologies and current attitudes

This can be demonstrated by looking at the theoretical ideology of nursing and comparing it with current attitudes towards nursing and nurses.

Nursing is concerned with nurturing or caring. This is fundamental to human life and growth, and is therefore highly valuable. If this was reflected upon, nurses would fiercely hang on to this basis of their role, and society would see it as being precious and worthy of status.

The reality is not so. The intimate physical care, or access to the person's private feelings and aspirations, inherent in all nursing acts, offers to the practitioner the opportunity of closeness between her/him and the client more than any other professional worker. Who else has the legitimate opportunity to strip someone of their clothes and wash their body, or to wipe someone's bottom after using the toilet? These intimate acts, and the opportunity for closeness, place the nurse in the unique position of being able to use and develop this closeness to therapeutic effect. Anyone can strip someone and immerse them in a tub of hot water — but to nurse is to do more than the simple physical act — it is to use that act to get closer to someone and promote healing. In reality, a belief in the importance of this has been lost by nurses and society. Intimate physical care is seen as 'basic nursing', unskilled, and rejected as lowly by qualified nurses who say that they did not train for three years to bath people. So it is delegated to the untrained auxiliary or nursing student.

Care-oriented specialties, such as geriatrics, long-term care, and district nursing, where this sort of work predominates, have much less status than cure-orientated specialties where high-tech medical work predominates. Nurses and the public want a high ratio of nurses in such areas, and a high ratio of auxiliaries in areas where intimate physical care predominates. It is difficult to recruit nurses to work in the so-called low-tech specialties.

So, the need for nurturing and intimate care which gives rise to the need for nursing is contradicted and denied.

Nursing is a basic human response. Nursing is a basic human response to a human need which transcends gender or age. People of all ages and sex need it, professionals of all ages and sex can be educated to practice. If this impulse is reflected upon, nurses would see the potential to nurse as being inherent in a large number of people, and the public would see a desire to nurse as one inherent in human beings. Again, the reality is not so. The intuitive desire to nurse is seen as one which is planted in the female at birth; the ability is aligned with being female, and males who choose to do it are less than male, are odd, or there is something wrong with them. Men in nursing, according to recent reports, cannot wait to get out of it and climb into work which manages nurses, or teaches them. So the idea that the potential to nurse can arise in any human being is contradicted and denied.

Nursing is difficult, skilled, and needs knowledge. This must be seen by us all as important, otherwise we would not have acts of Parliament which regulate entry to a register of nurses, and demand a standard period of education and training. Nursing is an intelligent occupation, says our theoretical ideology, because it uses practitioners who know more than the lay carer. Once again, the reality denies this. The general public, according to reports in the PINC campaign (public image of the nurse) and those snippets in the synapse column of the *Nursing Times*, see nurses as nice–kind–not needing much basic education — as simply carrying out the doctors' instructions. Clinical nurses may say that nursing is a skilled occupation, and may emphasise what a terrific responsibility is carried by the nurse, yet they too share those views of the public. They continue for example, to argue that a nursing auxiliary can be as good as a nurse; they criticise the rising entry requirements for entry on to nursing courses. They jibe at nurses who have studied to degree level, and for the whole of this century have vociferously opposed the conversion of the course of basic training from one which is educationally unsound, offers little intellectual stimulation, and gives a disgracefully sparse knowledge base to the student, into an educationally planned and tailored course designed to give the student the ability to think, and the opportunity to acquire the knowledge and skills that are needed by the nurse.

In our society work which is important and seen as skilled, such as doctoring, teaching, lawyering or engineering, demands a good educationally based preparation. This is not so for nursing.

So, the idea that work as important as nursing requires a high level of knowledge and skill is still contradicted and denied.

Nursing demands a degree of professionalism. Nursing *is* a profession. This is asserted both by our society and by nurses themselves. Nursing is usually referred to as the 'nursing profession', and nurses themselves refer to their occupational group as 'the profession'. It has to be said, however, that the notion of profession has both an attractive and unattractive side. Many argue that professionalisation is a means by which occupations can achieve exclusivity and power, that the established professions of today are elitist, and their excessive power is of no real benefit to society. When the general public, and nurses, constantly refer to nursing as a profession they are not really talking about this worrying side of professionalism, taking the word 'profession' in the sense of nursing having a commitment to service, a code of ethics or behaviour, and a recognised need for knowledge acquired through education. Nurses argue that they are professionals, and ask for the status and remuneration that goes with such an attribute. Positive professionalism implies that nurses will see their work as a little more than performing a series of tasks for eight hours a day; they will be concerned about the service they provide, and thus continually strive to gain new knowledge through evaluation or research, keeping aware of current advances in the discipline, and be personally accountable to the client for their actions.

The reality is again different. The large bulk of clinical nurses see themselves as people who perform a series of tasks for eight hours a day; they ask for policies and procedure books; on the one hand, they decry nurse management, but on the other they expect to be protected when something goes wrong, by passing the buck. A dismal number of nurses read the nursing journals, and even less are fully conversant with a code of ethics, or are even aware of the bodies that compile them. There is still confusion on the roles of the GNC, the UKCC, the national boards and the RCN. And the bulk of clinical nurses would not attend a course, meeting or seminar in their own time — keeping up to date is seen as the responsibility of management to provide in working hours.

So the idea that the positive values of a profession should be inherent in nursing is contradicted and denied.

These four major issues which, to my mind, made up the impulse that led to the formation of modern professional nursing are, whether we like it or not, vital to the future of clinical nursing as we know it. If we continue to lose sight of them, then nursing will die and be replaced by another occupation.

The opposition to a new era of nursing

The changes in our society over the last few hundred years have led to a devaluing of nursing, and this has influenced the socialisation of nurses in training. The worship of science, and growth in sexism, represent the major opposition to changes in nursing.

Objective, mechanistic science is now our new religion. We only believe in scientific facts, even though we know that it does little to explain us and the world. Because of this worship, all things scientific and mechanistic are afforded high status. People who work largely in a scientific way are important, and need to be given power and education. Less scientific, human kinds of work have less importance. They are — apparently — simple, need less education, status and power. This has had an overwhelming effect on how we view nursing. While the drive to be more scientific in nursing is important, its current obsessive nature is obscuring its true nature.

Linked with this rising of the scientific era is the growth in the belief that objectivity and the scientific mind are essentially masculine in nature, and that they are attributes usually found in men, whereas the softer, gentler, more human character is more often found in women. The domination of society by men has thus led to society affording more status and power to that which is scientific, and so to devaluing human skills, knowledge and work. But in nursing's current drive to gain power, it is attempting to make it both more scientific, and more like men's work.

Nurses themselves largely ignore these issues. This may be partly due to what White (1986) describes as factionalism in nursing. She argues in her analysis of the growth of nursing since the establishment of the National Health Service, that two factions of nurses exist, and that it is wrong to assume that nursing is united. One faction she describes as the *specialists*: nurses who are committed to developing nursing as a service; who are up to date; who want to be accountable to their clients; and who value education and reform. The second faction she calls the proletariat, or the *generalists*: they see nursing as a job of work; pay little attention to nursing as a national group; and identify on a parochial level with the hospital or base where they work. The latter faction predominates at the clinical level and pays lip service to the nursing impulse, but in reality denies it. The specialists, however, identify strongly with a national notion of nursing, and argue for the preservation of the nursing impulse. Unless more clinical nurses look outside their own ward or patch, and focus on the nursing impulse, it will remain hidden.

Kramer (1974) also describes four types of trained nurse: the rutter, the lateral arabesquer, the organisation woman, and the bicultural trouble-maker. She argues that when a nurse finishes training she or he becomes one of these. The *rutter* quickly takes on the values of the people with whom she works, and thinks about little concerning nursing on a wider scale. The *lateral arabesquer* is disappointed with the reality of nursing, moves from one role to another, and usually leaves clinical nursing practice; the *organisation woman* climbs the hierarchy and identifies more with the goals and rules of the organisation rather than with the true goals of nursing; the *bicultural trouble-maker* hangs on to this true nature, dislikes the system where it is suppressed, and stays to try and change things. Thus, the rutter and the bicultural trouble-maker often stay in clinical nursing. Whilst the rutter plods on maintaining the status quo, the bicultural trouble-maker does the job, and rocks the boat in order to uphold her beliefs in nursing. In the process, the rutter has an easy, comfortable life, whilst the bicultural trouble-maker faces hostility and unpopularity (usually seen as a 'good nurse', but boy, she's trouble!). It would seem that we have far too *many* rutters and far too *few* bicultural trouble-makers.

Despite the desire in nursing to maintain the status quo, and the outside pressures that it encourages to do so, evidence from other countries and experience in the nursing units suggest that primary nursing and the units' application of it offers benefits to patients, is cost-effective, and is satisfying and acceptable to health care workers.

BENEFITS TO THE PATIENTS

Patients nursed in a nurse-oriented environment that values the individual and views him/her as a whole person are more independent, more satisfied with care, and more socially active (Hall *et al.*, 1975; Pearson, 1985). The quality of care in an American inpatient unit that adopted primary nursing was found to be significantly higher using the Quality of Patient Care Scale (Qualpacs; Wandelt and Ager, 1976) than in units that used a team nursing approach (Steckel, Barnfather and Owens, 1980). Marram (1980), in a review of research studies on the subject, reports that primary nursing results in: 'fewer omissions in care, higher quality nursing performance . . . more personalised, individualised care as reported by patients'.

Studies in the United States of a unit focusing on nursing as a therapy suggest that placing a high value on nursing rather than medical technology improves the patient's quality of life, leads to a lower readmission rate, and is seen as a highly valued service by both doctors and patient. In this American unit (the Loeb Center for Nursing) nursing is seen as a therapy in itself, in that nurturing, befriending and giving intimate physical care can be as powerful a healing force as the initial medical care and just as skilled and dependent upon a social knowledge base acquired through professional education if not more. The nursing units at Burford and Oxford are based on this philosophy.

139

I believe that there is an increasing need for this kind of nursing in our society. Currently medicine and medical technology, supported by nursing, offer great benefits to many patients but are inappropriate for many more. The primary health needs of many people are for teaching, for rehabilitation and for the healing and growth that flows from the person being cared for as a whole person. Many of these are currently occupying NHS beds which are, of necessity, directing most energy towards intervention to relieve biological crises. Nursing has the potential, but has not yet demonstrated the ability, to help provide an alternative type of care as serious biological crises are resolved.

The rapid growth of effective medicine since the 1940s has dominated the way in which nursing has developed. Nursing has followed on medical advances — as has the whole development of the National Health Service. Medical specialties depend greatly on qualified nurses, and nurse training has been directed towards providing nurses for these new specialties rather than to the skilled nursing that patients need, regardless of their medical diagnosis.

This lack of attention to the fundamental technology of nursing is reflected in the education of nurses. There is as yet (1987) no common education in nursing as a discipline; nurses can only train for specialist registers. Post-basic nursing education, where it has been developed, mainly reflects medical specialisation rather than the elements of advanced clinical nursing.

Since the publication of the Report on Senior Nursing Staff Structure (Salmon Committee, Ministry of Health, 1966) and the reorganisation of the health service in 1974 and 1982, nursing has been more concerned with the management of nursing services than with the development of clinical nursing. This orientation has been influenced by forces outside nursing and in particular by government. Nursing has therefore responded largely reactively over the last 40 years.

There are now signs that nursing is developing an independent view from within its ranks and is trying to respond more directly to the changing needs of patients. This nursing view has been influenced by the university departments of nursing. The Department of Nursing at the University of Manchester has particularly influenced thinking about nursing as a therapy in its own right, with its holistic approach and seeing the patient as an equal partner in his/her own nursing care. The academic nursing departments, however, are usually impotent in testing and applying their thinking, which is the whole purpose of a practice discipline such as nursing or medicine, because they have no patients; they have no clinical audits.

Creating nursing beds in nursing units could become more than a badly needed service for clients — it could also provide a creative practice base for developing a new technology.

In 1983, when the Loeb Center proposed setting up such a unit where all direct care was given by registered nurses, based on the 'case' method traditional only in district nursing, it was seen as revolutionary, and it is still seen in that light today. The basis of practice in a nursing unit encompasses the current trends in this country towards the use of the nursing process — patient allocation, holism, and all the other 'in' things — but it concentrates on the nurses working with the patient, with each other, and with other disciplines, in peer rather than hierarchical relationships.

Nurses in such units have to learn the most important truth — that patients are the achievers, and that nurses are the facilitators, teachers, supporters and nurturers (Hall *et al.*, 1975). They need to appreciate that there is nothing simple about patients, who are complex human beings, or a nurse who is also complex and who finds herself involved in the complex helping relationship.

The exclusive aspect of nursing is the nurturing one: it provides the opportunity for closeness; it necessitates seeing the process as essentially an interpersonal relationship. This *close personal process* takes in the intimate bodily care of patients: bathing, feeding, toileting, dressing, undressing, positioning and moving. This nurturing aspect involves the laying on of hands with *comfort* of the patient the main interest and, if understood, the main result. It is not, however, the unskilled intuitive feminine acts of a mother — but highly skilled, goal-oriented, and based on sound knowledge.

The nurse who knows herself/himself can also like and trust the patient enough to work *with* him professionally, rather than *for* him. In this way the nurse recognises that the power to heal lies in the *patient* and not in the nurse. She/he takes satisfaction and pride in the ability to help the patient use this source of power to grow and develop, and becomes comfortable working together with members of other professions.

141

The nature of nursing in relation to nursing beds is thus rooted in the nurse as nurturer, teacher, facilitator and friend, using a technology appropriate to nursing. Nursing beds could become places to admit patients who no longer, or perhaps did not originally, need medical intervention leading to cure, but who need nursing leading to healing. Such a provision in the NHS would serve to both develop the technology of nursing, and to demonstrate its effectiveness to the world.

The technology of clinical nursing in the year 2000 may be hi-tech, medically related and unrecognisable to us, with comforting and nurturing delegated to a lower occupational group. Or will it be a more highly developed form of the sort of nursing we are now trying to achieve? If we wish this to be so, there really is an urgent need to convince policy-makers and the consumers of health care that nursing heals — but I fear that society and its number-crunching, objective leaders will continue to overvalue hi-tech and devalue the 'human-tech' of nursing.

THE COSTS

Critics of this new era of nursing focus on its cost-effectiveness. The nursing units appear to demonstrate that they are in fact cost-effective. Therapeutic nursing generates costs in two areas — financial and personal.

Financial

Staffing and running costs in both units are less than in comparable units in the district. This is largely because staffing is based on the belief that people in hospital need access to a qualified nurse 24 hours a day, and that one nurse can be reasonably expected to care for up to eight patients in a subacute unit. Thus, two nurses are on duty throughout the day and night. This contrasts with higher numbers of nurses on duty in areas where a 'mixed' team is the norm. For example, the majority of hospital wards tend to have an average of six nursing staff on duty in a morning, often consisting of one to two trained nurses and four to five students or nursing auxiliaries. In addition, domestic staff are on duty, but they are not accountable to the nurse and thus their work pattern cannot be controlled by ward staff. In the 16 bed nursing unit, two nurses are on duty in the morning, supported by two care assistants and one ward coordinator. While all direct care is given by the registered nurses, activities which do not involve patients directly are performed by the care assistants and coordinator. The registered nurses (who have the highest salary) are freed to nurse, but also have the authority to direct the support staff.

In 1986, the Oxford unit had staffing costs which were 25 per cent lower than any comparable wards in the health district, and the Burford unit's costs were 10 per cent lower. Because of its small size, Burford's costs are likely to be higher than units which form part of a large hospital, as there resources such as catering and portering can be 'pooled'. Despite this, costs were lower than other subacute units. (For the purposes of this discussion, subacute refers to areas where patients require a high level of care, but who do not undergo intensive medical investigations or procedures.) Acute areas, such as surgical wards, have been found to require a ratio of one registered nurse to five to six patients (Brown, 1980), plus support staff, when primary nursing is used. Such ratios are still likely to be less costly than the current approach of using 'mixed teams'.

Support staff, unlike nursing auxiliaries, are not employed as nurses, so are considerably cheaper to employ. They are, however, more expensive than domestic staff in terms of salary, but sickness and absence levels are lower because there is greater job satisfaction when support workers both clean the environment *and* assist nurses directly when requested to do so. Experience in both units shows clearly that: reducing the number of nurses on duty, but increasing the quality of nurse (that is, only employing qualified nurses); increasing the number of support staff (such as care assistants and ward coordinators); broadening the role of support staff; and making support staff accountable to nurses all lead to less costs, a more effective service, and greater job satisfaction for both nurses and support staff.

Changing staff structures in this way is, however, extremely difficult because it challenges tradition and meets considerable resistance. Current thinking on staffing methods in Britain, as reflected in major reports, reflects the desire to maintain mixed teams of carers, and to reject the logical argument that professional nursing in hospitals should be given by professional nurses. In a document which attempts to rationalise nurse education in the United Kingdom, the United Kingdom Central Council for Nursing, Midwifery and Health Visiting (UKCC, 1986) argues that nursing auxiliaries should be phased out of nursing service, and that a new assistant grade be introduced, known as an 'aide'. While suggesting that the term 'nursing' or 'nurse' should not be prefixed to the title of an assistant, the report fails to assert that, in fact, an assistant nurse is not needed. Care assistants in the nursing unit are seen as generic assistants who are primarily concerned with domestic work, freeing nurses to nurse. The proposed aide, however, is distinct from domestic service workers, and therefore likely to assume the status of an assistant nurse once established. Thus, the notion that all care should be given by registered nurses is practically addressed in this report. Interestingly, the report also demands that students of nursing should cease to be regarded as service providers, yet it still foresees a need for assistants. Nursing in the western world seems to be obsessed with the view that an all-qualified nursing service is either unnecessary or impractical, and that a team of mixed workers can best serve patients needs. The Department of Health and Social Security in the United Kingdom commissioned work on 'skill mix' to try and identify norms in a variety of specialties (DHSS, 1986). The report discovered a number of interesting findings. In long-stay wards with low staffing levels, and low ratios of qualified to unqualified nurses, it was found that 'only the basic physical needs of the patients were being met'. They also found that 'gaps in the support provided by the paramedical services were invariably filled by the nursing staff' and 'inadequate clerical and domestic services sometimes deflected nursing staff from direct patient care'.

However, the main thrust of the report was on determining the best skill mix and devising ways of rationalising it nationwide, rather than on addressing the issue of skill mix in itself. The work in the nursing development units suggests that the term 'skill mix' is inappropriate when discussing the provision of skilled nursing in hospitals. *All* patients deserve skilled nursing; *all* nursing should be given by skilled nurses; and the only way to be sure that a nurse is skilled is through providing professional training and regulating practice through registration. 'Skill mix' is not a concept applied in the practice of medicine, or teaching, or other skilled occupations, yet it is still

144

held up as reasonable in nursing. The DHSS (1986) report found that the majority of senior nurses favoured mixed teams in that they saw that '. . . given the right environment and adequate training and supervision, nursing auxiliaries and assistants had a useful role in the delivery of patient care'.

Personal

The initial reaction of many nurses to the notion of primary nursing and the philosophy of the nurse becoming involved in the life of the patient is to suggest that this is too stressful and that the personal costs for the nurse are too high. In the early stages of introducing this work method in the units, open expressions of emotion and apparent stress from nurses were evident. Further exploration suggests, however, that the atmosphere of the unit does encourage openness, but does not in itself increase the stress inherent in looking after people who are ill, in pain, or vulnerable. Indeed, many nurses now feel that primary nursing and acting therapeutically are in fact less stressful than practising in a traditional style which demands detachment, conformity to routines, and a clouding of the opportunity to be responsible for one's own work. Our conclusion at this stage is that the personal costs are no higher than any other approach to the delivery of nursing care, and may well, in the final analysis, be less.

CONCLUSIONS

If 'basis' nursing as described in this book is now outmoded and outdated, then we are going along the right road to shed it. But if the need for nurturing, comforting and healing gives rise to the need for nursing, then nursing has to do something.

First, it has to convince society of the truism that the less objective and scientific areas of work are as important as the scientific. Neither has supremacy. At the same time, it has to be convinced *itself* that the nurturing aspect of nursing is as skilled and knowledge-based as the high-tech aspect.

Second, it has to convince itself, and society, that the nursing impulse is not a female, mother-nature-endowed personality trait. Neither should it try and become more scientific, and therefore men's work. It must become *people's* work which is equal to that of other work.

Third, nursing must try to both recruit more people who will be like White's specialists, or Kramer's bicultural trouble-makers, and ensure that the educational course designed to produce a nurse preserves these abilities, rather than suppresses them.

The basis of nursing that made it emerge as an occupation stems from the fundamental human need for nurturing. Most clinical nurses pay lip service to it, but continue to deny it. Society follows suit. If nursing is to survive and continue to meet this fundamental need in society, it needs to reflect on its basic core.

Styles (1977) says:

In the beginning, God created nursing.
He (or She) said, I will take a solid, simple
   significant system of education and an adequate,
   applicable base of clinical research, and
On these rocks, will I build My greatest gift
   to mankind — nursing practice.
On the seventh day, He threw up his hands
And has left it up to us.

The future of practical, hands-on nursing obviously lies in the hands of clinical nurses — who need to assert the potential of nursing as a means of healing.

REFERENCES

Brown, B. (1980) 'Leadership on the Primary Nursing Unit'. *Nursing Dimensions*, 9, 13–17.
DHSS (1986) *Mix and Match: A Review of Nursing Skill Mix*. (DHSS, London).
Hall, L.E., Alfano, G.J., Rifkin, M. and Levine, H.S. (1975) *Longitudinal Effects of an Experimental Nursing Process*. (Loeb Center for Nursing, New York).
Kitson, A. (1984) 'Steps towards the identification and development of nursing therapeutic function in the care of the hospital elderly', *unpublished PhD thesis*. (University of Ulster, Coleraine).
Kramer, M. (1974) *Reality Shock*. (C.V. Mosby, St Louis).
Marram van Servellem, G. (1980) 'Evaluating the Impact of Primary Nursing: Outcomes'. *Nursing Dimensions*, 9, 48–51.

Pearson, A. (1983) *The Clinical Nursing Unit*. (Heinemann, London).

Pearson, A. (1985) 'Introducing New Norms in a Nursing Unit and an Analysis of the Process of Change', *unpublished PhD thesis*, Department of Social Science and Administration, University of London, Goldsmiths College.

Pearson, A., Morris, P. and Whitehouse, C. (1985) 'Consumer Oriented Groups: a New Approach to Inter-disciplinary Teaching'. *Journal of the Royal College of General Practitioners*, 35, 301–383.

Pembrey, S. (1985) 'A Framework for Care . . . One Level of Nurse'. *Nursing Times*, 81(50), 47–9.

Robinson, V. (1946) *White Caps: The Story of Nursing*. (J.B. Lippincott, Philadelphia).

Royal College of Nursing (1979) *Discussion Paper of the Working Party of a Clinical Career Structure for Nurses*. (RCN, London).

Royal College of Nursing (1981) *Towards Standards*. (RCN, London).

Salmon Committee, Ministry of Health (1966) *Report on Senior Nursing Staff Structure*. (HMSO, London).

Steckel, S.B., Barnfather, J. and Owens, M. (1980) 'Implementing Primary Nursing Within a Research Design'. *Nursing Dimensions*, 9, 78–81.

Styles, M. (1977) 'Doctoral Education in Nursing; the Current Situation in Historical Perspective', in *National Conference on Doctoral Education in Nursing*. (University of Pennsylvania, Philadelphia).

United Kingdom Central Council for Nursing, Midwifery and Health Visiting (1983) *Code of Professional Conduct for the Nurse, Midwife and Health Visitor*. (UKCC, London).

United Kingdom Central Council for Nursing, Midwifery and Health Visiting (1986) *Project 2000*, (UKCC, London).

Wandelt, M.A. and Ager, J. (1976) *Quality Patient Care Scale*, (Wayne State University Press, Ohio).

White, R. (1986) *The Effects of the NHS on the Nursing Profession 1948–1961*. (Kings Fund, London).

Index